EXECUTIVE FUNCTIONING WORKBOOK FOR KIDS AGES 7 – 11

44 PROVEN ACTIVITIES TO HELP KIDS WITH TIME MANAGEMENT, IMPULSE CONTROL, FOCUS, AND EMOTIONAL REGULATION AT HOME AND SCHOOL.

A. E. NICHOLLS

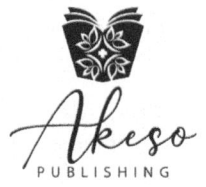

Copyright © 2024 Akeso Publishing. All rights reserved.

The content within this book may not be reproduced, duplicated, or transmitted without direct written permission from the author or the publisher.

Under no circumstances will any blame or legal responsibility be held against the publisher, or author, for any damages, reparation, or monetary loss due to the information contained within this book, either directly or indirectly.

Legal Notice:

This book is copyright protected. It is only for personal use. You cannot amend, distribute, sell, use, quote, or paraphrase any part of the content within this book, without the consent of the author or publisher.

Disclaimer Notice:

Please note the information contained within this document is for educational and entertainment purposes only. All effort has been expended to present accurate, up-to-date, reliable, and complete information. No warranties of any kind are declared or implied. Readers acknowledge that the author is not engaged in the rendering of legal, financial, medical, or professional advice. The content within this book has been derived from various sources. Please consult a licensed professional before attempting any techniques outlined in this book.

By reading this document, the reader agrees that under no circumstances is the author responsible for any losses, direct or indirect, that are incurred as a result of the use of the information contained within this document, including, but not limited to, errors, omissions, or inaccuracies.

To the tireless parents and caregivers nurturing young minds:
Your love and dedication inspire this work. May these pages support you in your incredible journey.

To my amazing occupational therapy clients:
Your resilience, curiosity, and joy continue to inspire me every day. This book is a testament to your boundless potential.

May you always know that you are capable of amazing things. Keep exploring, learning, and growing.

With love and admiration,

A.E. Nicholls

CONTENTS

Introduction   ix

1. Understanding Executive Functioning   1
2. Enhancing Focus and Concentration   9
3. Improving Instruction-Following Skills   24
4. Emotional Regulation Techniques   38
5. Time Management Strategies   52
6. Enhancing Memory Skills   66
   A Moment for Reflection   81
7. Developing Flexible Thinking   83
8. Building Social Skills   98
9. Enhancing Self-Control   112
10. Problem-Solving Skills   126
11. Encouraging Self-Reflection   140
12. Parental Involvement and Support   154

Afterword   169
A Final Note of Gratitude   171
Bibliography   173
Also by A. E. Nicholls   177

HOW TO GET THE MOST OUT OF THIS BOOK

PRINTABLE | FULL COLOR
ACTIVITY WORKSHEETS

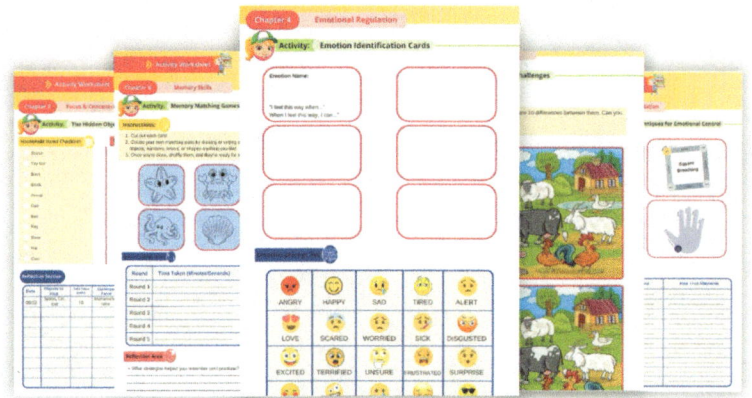

INSTANT - PRINTABLE - UNLIMITED - DOWNLOAD

To help your child with their executive functioning journey, we have created free downloads of all 44 full-color activity worksheets to help make learning fun and effective.

Please print as many as you need. They aren't just tasks to complete but opportunities for your child to develop essential life skills.

Please use the link or QR code below.
https://akeso-publishing.ck.page/9083dc556f

INTRODUCTION

"Parents are the ultimate role models for children. Every word, movement, and action has an effect. No other person or outside force has a greater influence on a child than the parent."

— BOB KEESHAN

Sarah, a bright and curious nine-year-old, often finds herself overwhelmed by her daily school routine. She struggles to keep track of her assignments, forgets to turn in her homework, and frequently loses her belongings. At home, her parents notice her becoming frustrated easily, having trouble focusing on tasks, and experiencing meltdowns over seemingly minor issues. For Sarah's parents, these challenges are both heartbreaking and exhausting. They want to help but feel unsure where to start.

Stories like Sarah's are common. Many children face difficulties with skills that seem straightforward: managing their time, controlling impulses, staying focused, and regulating their emotions. These are known as executive functioning skills. Just like an orchestra needs a conductor to organize and direct the musicians, children need strong executive functioning skills to help them manage their thoughts, actions, and emotions.

Executive functioning skills are the mental processes that enable us to plan, focus attention, remember instructions, and juggle multiple tasks successfully. They help children with tasks such as organizing their schoolwork, following multi-step directions, and managing their emotions during social interactions. When these skills are underdeveloped, children can struggle in both academic settings and everyday life.

The significance of these skills becomes even more apparent when we consider the statistics. Research shows that approximately 10-15% of children are diagnosed with ADHD, a condition closely linked to executive functioning challenges. Moreover, many neurodiverse children, including those with autism spectrum disorder, also experience difficulties in these areas. These statistics highlight a pressing need for effective strategies to support children in developing their executive functioning skills.

My name is Amy Nicholls, and for over a decade, I have worked as a pediatric occupational therapist. My passion lies in helping children develop the life skills they need to thrive. My approach is holistic, recognizing that each child is unique and requires a tailored strategy to support their growth. As a parent myself, I understand the complexities and rewards of guiding children through their developmental stages. This book is a culmination of my experience and dedication, designed to provide parents with practical tools to support their children.

The purpose of this book is clear: to help children improve their executive functioning skills through actionable and engaging activities. Whether your child is neurotypical or neurodiverse, the strategies and exercises in this book are designed to be accessible and effective. We focus on key areas such as time management, impulse control, focus, and emotional regulation. These skills are crucial for success in both school and everyday life, and they can be developed with the right support and practice.

What sets this book apart is its emphasis on practical, hands-on activities. You won't find confusing metaphors or overly complex language here. Instead, each activity is clearly explained and easy to implement. The goal is to make these exercises as engaging, straightforward, and as fun as possible so you and your child can work on them together without feeling overwhelmed.

The structure of the book is designed to guide you step-by-step with activity worksheets at the end of each chapter. We begin with activities to improve focus and attention, such as the "Hidden Object Concentration Game," which helps children practice sustained attention in a fun and interactive way. Next, we move on to exercises for emotional regulation, like "Emotion Charades," where children learn to identify and express their feelings. Time management skills are addressed through activities like "The Homework Planner," which helps children break down tasks and manage their time effectively. Finally, we cover social skills with activities that promote positive interactions and communication.

To enhance your child's learning experience, we've made an exciting addition to our resources. We've created free downloads of all 44 full-color activity worksheets. These vibrant, printable sheets are designed to make learning fun and effective for your child. You can access and print a new schedule every week or print as many of the worksheets as you need using the QR code below.

Throughout the book, the tone is supportive, practical, and engaging. I want you to feel empowered as a parent, knowing that you have effective tools at your disposal. Your involvement is crucial. The activities are designed to be collaborative, fostering a strong parent-child relationship. By working together, you can help your child develop the skills they need to navigate their world with confidence and resilience.

In summary, this book is not just a collection of activities; it is a resource to help you understand and support your child's development. By focusing on practical strategies and encouraging a collaborative approach, we can make a meaningful difference in your child's life. Thank you for joining me on this journey. Let's get started and help your child reach their fullest potential.

1

UNDERSTANDING EXECUTIVE FUNCTIONING

"Parenting a child with executive functioning challenges requires patience, creativity, and resilience. Remember, every step you take to support your child is a step toward their success and independence."

— PEG DAWSON

One morning, Emma was trying to get her seven-year-old son, Jack, ready for school. Despite multiple reminders, Jack forgot to pack his homework, couldn't find his shoes, and ended up in tears because he lost track of time and missed breakfast. Emma felt frustrated and helpless. She knew Jack was bright and capable, but something was clearly getting in his way.

These everyday struggles can feel overwhelming for both parents and children. Many kids face challenges with executive functioning skills, which are essential for managing oneself and one's resources. These skills include time management, impulse control, focus, and emotional regulation.

1.1 WHAT ARE EXECUTIVE FUNCTIONING SKILLS?

Executive functioning skills are cognitive processes that enable us to plan, focus attention, remember instructions, and juggle multiple tasks successfully. These skills are often likened to the brain's control center, managing how we organize and respond to information. They include working memory, flexible thinking, and impulse control. These skills are essential for daily functions and academic success, helping children complete tasks, follow directions, and manage their emotions.

Working memory is the ability to hold information in mind while using it. For instance, a child using working memory can remember the steps in a math problem while solving it. Flexible thinking allows children to adjust to new situations and solve problems creatively. This skill helps them adapt when plans change or when they need to think of different ways to approach a task. Impulse control is the ability to manage immediate reactions and stay focused. It helps children wait their turn, follow rules, and think before acting.

Consider a child named Lucas who struggles with working memory. During math class, he often forgets the steps to solve multi-step problems, even though he understands the concept. His teacher notices that Lucas frequently leaves parts of his math problems incomplete, not because he doesn't know the answer but because he forgets the process midway. Another example is Sophie, who has difficulty with flexible thinking. When her teacher announces a change in the classroom routine, Sophie becomes anxious and disruptive, unable to adapt to the new plan.

Understanding these skills is crucial for parents as it helps identify specific challenges their child may be facing. By recognizing these difficulties, parents can better support their child's development and find effective strategies to help them succeed. For instance, knowing that a child struggles with impulse control can lead to implementing activities that teach self-regulation and patience, providing a more supportive environment for learning and growth.

VISUAL AID: EXECUTIVE FUNCTIONING SKILLS CHECKLIST

Working Memory:

- Can your child remember multi-step instructions?
- Does your child complete tasks that require holding information in mind?
- Can your child follow a sequence of events or steps?

Flexible Thinking:

- How does your child react to changes in routine?
- Can your child find different ways to solve a problem?
- Is your child able to adapt to new situations?

Impulse Control:

- Does your child wait their turn during games or activities?
- Can your child follow rules without constant reminders?
- How does your child handle frustration or excitement?

These questions can help you identify areas where your child may need additional support. Recognizing these challenges is the first step in empowering your child to develop stronger executive functioning skills.

Understanding and supporting your child's executive functioning skills can transform their daily experiences. These skills are the foundation for managing tasks, controlling impulses, and adapting to new situations. By focusing on practical strategies and engaging activities, we can help children like Jack, Lucas, and Sophie navigate their world with confidence and resilience.

1.2 THE IMPORTANCE OF EXECUTIVE FUNCTIONING IN DAILY LIFE

Imagine the typical morning routine: the alarm goes off, and it's time to get ready for school. For many children, this involves getting dressed, brushing their teeth, eating breakfast, and packing their school bag. Each of these tasks requires a certain level of executive functioning. Time management helps them complete each task promptly, while impulse control stops them from getting distracted by toys or the TV. Focus is needed to remember each step, and emotional regulation helps them stay calm and on track. When these skills are underdeveloped, mornings can become chaotic, leading to stress for both the child and the parents.

The school day itself is full of executive functioning challenges. Completing homework assignments, for instance, demands sustained attention and the ability to break tasks into manageable steps. A child with strong executive functioning can plan their homework time, stay focused on the task at hand, and turn in complete assignments on time. In contrast, a child struggling with these skills might find it hard to start their homework, forget part of the assignment, or get sidetracked by distractions. This can lead to incomplete work, missed deadlines, and frustration.

Participation in social activities and group work also hinges on strong executive functioning skills. Whether it's a team project or a game on the playground, children need to manage their emotions, communicate effectively, and adapt to changing dynamics. A child who struggles with impulse control might interrupt peers or have difficulty sharing, leading to conflicts. Those who find it hard to manage their emotions may have frequent outbursts, making it tough to maintain friendships. These skills are not just academic; they are crucial for social success and emotional well-being.

In the classroom, executive functioning skills are pivotal for academic success. Following classroom instructions requires the ability to listen, remember, and execute multiple steps. This is particularly true during complex tasks or when instructions are given verbally. A child with strong working memory can hold these instructions in mind and act on them, while a child with weaker skills might forget key steps, leading to incomplete or incorrect work. Completing and turning in homework on time also relies on these skills. It involves planning, time management, and the ability to stay organized. Without these skills, children may struggle to keep track of assignments, leading to lower grades and increased stress.

Test-taking is another area where executive functioning skills come into play. During tests, children need to manage their time wisely, stay focused, and recall information accurately. Those who can regulate their emotions are less likely to be overwhelmed by test anxiety, allowing them to perform at their best. Effective test-taking strategies, such as skimming questions before answering or double-checking work, also rely on strong executive functioning.

Emotional regulation is another critical aspect influenced by executive functioning skills. Managing emotions during stressful situations, like a disagreement with a friend or a challenging school task, requires the ability to stay calm and think clearly. Children who can regulate their emotions are better equipped to handle frustration, disappointment, and even excitement. This emotional stability allows them to navigate social interactions smoothly and maintain positive relationships with peers and adults.

Effective communication is another area where executive functioning skills are essential. Children need to listen, process information, and respond appropriately. This is particularly important during group activities or collaborative projects, where clear and respectful communication is key. Being able to express thoughts and feelings clearly helps children build stronger connections and resolve conflicts more effectively.

It's important for parents to understand these skills. Observing a child's daily routines and identifying signs of executive functioning challenges can provide valuable insights. For instance, frequent forgetfulness, difficulty following multi-step instructions, or emotional outbursts during transitions might indicate areas where support is needed. Implementing daily routines that support skill development can make a significant difference. Simple strategies like visual schedules, checklists, and regular practice of mindfulness can help children strengthen these skills over time.

By focusing on these areas, parents can provide the support their children need to succeed academically, socially, and emotionally.

1.3 EXECUTIVE FUNCTIONING CHALLENGES IN NEURODIVERSE KIDS

Neurodiversity is a term that acknowledges and respects the diverse ways in which human brains can function. It includes conditions such as ADHD (Attention Deficit Hyperactivity Disorder) and autism spectrum disorder (ASD), which are characterized by unique patterns of thinking and behavior. These conditions often affect executive functioning skills, leading to a variety of challenges. Neurodiverse children may experience differences in how they manage tasks, regulate emotions, and interact with others. The variation in executive functioning challenges among these children is significant, making it crucial to understand and address their specific needs.

Children with ADHD often struggle with impulse control and emotional regulation. For example, they might find it difficult to stay seated during class, leading to frequent interruptions and a hard time focusing on lessons. In contrast, children with autism may have trouble adapting to changes in their routines, causing anxiety and resistance when faced with new situations. These children might also struggle to maintain focus and attention, become easily overwhelmed by sensory stimuli, or have rigid thinking patterns that make flexible problem-solving challenging.

Consider a child with ADHD who can't stay seated during class. This child might frequently get up, fidget, or talk out of turn, disrupting not only their own learning but also the learning environment for others. Their struggle with impulse control makes it hard for them to follow classroom rules, leading to frequent reprimands and a negative self-image. Another example is a child with autism who finds it hard to adapt to a new school routine. The sudden change in schedule can cause extreme distress, resulting in meltdowns or withdrawal. This child's difficulty with flexible thinking makes it challenging to cope with transitions, creating a barrier to their academic and social success.

To support neurodiverse children, parents can implement several practical strategies. Visual schedules and reminders can provide a sense of structure and predictability, helping children know what to expect and reducing anxiety. For instance, a visual timetable showing each part of the school day can help a child with autism feel more secure and prepared for transitions. Using behavior charts and reward systems can also be effective. These tools reinforce positive behaviors and provide clear, consistent feedback. For a child with ADHD, a reward system that recognizes staying seated for a set period can motivate them to regulate their impulses better.

Mindfulness and relaxation exercises are another valuable strategy. These practices can help children develop better emotional regulation and focus. Simple activities like deep breathing, guided imagery, or yoga can be incorporated into daily routines. Encouraging a child to take a few minutes to breathe deeply before starting homework can help them calm their mind and prepare for focused work. Similarly, guided imagery, where a child imagines themselves in a calm and happy place, can provide a mental break and reduce stress.

Moreover, creating a supportive and understanding environment is crucial. Parents should recognize and celebrate small successes, understanding that progress may come in small steps. For example, if a child with ADHD manages to stay seated for a few minutes longer than usual, this achievement should be acknowledged and praised. Building a strong, positive relationship based on trust and encouragement can significantly impact a child's ability to develop their executive functioning skills.

Interactive tools can also be beneficial. For instance, a checklist that a child can physically check off as they complete tasks can provide a sense of accomplishment and help them stay organized. A reflection journal where children can write or draw about their feelings and experiences can also be a valuable tool for self-awareness and emotional regulation. These tools make the abstract concept of executive functioning more concrete and manageable for children.

I'll dive into activities soon, but understanding and addressing the unique executive functioning challenges faced by neurodiverse children requires patience, empathy, and a willingness to adapt. By implementing visual schedules, behavior charts, mindfulness exercises, and interactive tools, parents can provide the support needed to help their children thrive. Recognizing the diversity in how children think and behave is the first step towards creating an inclusive environment where every child can succeed.

1.4 STATISTICS AND REAL-LIFE EXAMPLES

Understanding the prevalence of executive functioning challenges in children is vital for grasping the scope of these issues. As mentioned briefly above, approximately 10-15% of children are diagnosed with ADHD, according to the Centers for Disease Control and Prevention (CDC). This statistic underscores the significant number of children who may struggle with executive functioning skills. Furthermore, research indicates that children with ADHD are often at a higher risk of academic difficulties, with many experiencing lower grades and higher dropout rates. Additionally, children with autism spectrum disorder (ASD) frequently encounter executive functioning challenges, particularly in areas requiring flexible thinking and impulse control. The social and emotional impacts are equally profound. Studies show that children with executive functioning difficulties often face higher levels of anxiety and depression, leading to strained peer relationships and reduced social engagement.

To illustrate how specific strategies can make a difference, let's consider the case of Ethan, a nine-year-old who struggled with focus and attention in school. Ethan's teachers noted that he had trouble staying on task and often appeared distracted. His parents decided to implement a structured plan that included regular breaks, visual schedules, and mindfulness exercises. Over several months, Ethan's ability to focus improved significantly. He began completing his assignments more consistently and showed greater engagement in class discussions. This case study highlights how targeted interventions can lead to meaningful improvements in a child's executive functioning skills.

Another example is the Garcia family, who successfully implemented time management techniques to help their daughter, Sofia, manage her daily routines more effectively. Sofia had difficulty transitioning between activities, often resulting in meltdowns and missed deadlines. The family introduced a visual timer and a daily checklist to help Sofia understand and manage her time better. They also established a consistent morning and evening routine. Within weeks, Sofia's ability to transition between tasks improved, and her overall stress levels decreased. The time management strategies not only made Sofia's daily life more manageable but also fostered a more harmonious family environment.

In the classroom, teachers play a crucial role in supporting children with executive functioning challenges. Mrs. Thompson, a fifth-grade teacher, incorporated executive functioning activities into her daily lessons. She used tools like graphic organizers, checklists, and collaborative projects to help her students develop planning and organizational skills. One of her students, Liam, who struggled with impulse control and focus, showed remarkable progress. By breaking down tasks into smaller, manageable steps and providing consistent feedback, Mrs. Thompson helped Liam stay on track and complete his assignments more efficiently. This example demonstrates the positive impact that structured, supportive teaching methods can have on children's executive functioning skills.

Success stories from parents further underscore the potential for improvement. One parent shared how their son, diagnosed with ADHD, made significant strides after participating in a structured program that included cognitive-behavioral therapy (CBT) and executive functioning coaching. The program taught him strategies for managing his impulses, staying organized, and improving his time management skills. As a result, his academic performance improved, and he became more confident in his abilities. Another parent highlighted their daughter's progress in emotional regulation after incorporating mindfulness exercises into their daily routine. The child learned to recognize and manage her emotions better, leading to fewer outbursts and improved relationships with her peers.

Improving executive functioning skills can have a broader impact on a child's overall development. Better academic performance is often the most visible outcome, as children become more organized, focused, and capable of handling complex tasks. However, the benefits extend beyond academics. Improved emotional well-being is another significant outcome. Children who develop strong executive functioning skills are better equipped to manage stress, handle setbacks, and regulate their emotions. This emotional stability contributes to a more positive self-image and greater resilience in the face of challenges.

Enhanced social interactions are another critical benefit. Children with well-developed executive functioning skills are more likely to communicate effectively, work collaboratively with peers, and build strong, healthy relationships. These social skills are essential for success in school and beyond, helping children navigate the complexities of social dynamics and fostering a sense of belonging and community.

In summary, understanding the prevalence and impact of executive functioning challenges is the first step in addressing these issues. Through case studies and success stories, we see the transformative potential of targeted strategies and interventions. By focusing on practical, engaging activities that support the development of executive functioning skills, we can help children achieve their fullest potential, both academically and socially, so let's get started!

2

ENHANCING FOCUS AND CONCENTRATION

"Focus and concentration can be developed through consistent practice and creating an environment that minimizes distractions."

— DANIEL GOLEMAN

When eight-year-old Mia found herself constantly distracted during her homework sessions, her mother, Lisa, decided to try something new. She introduced a simple game that not only captured Mia's attention but also seemed to improve her ability to concentrate over time. This game, which involved searching for hidden objects around the house, became a fun and effective way to help Mia build her focus. It was a game that could be adapted to different settings and tailored to various levels of difficulty, making it a versatile tool for enhancing concentration.

2.1 THE HIDDEN OBJECT CONCENTRATION GAME

The Hidden Object Concentration Game is designed to help children improve their attention span through a fun and interactive activity. By searching for objects hidden around a room, children practice sustained attention and develop their ability to focus on a task. The simplicity of the game makes it easy to set up and play in various settings, whether at home, in the classroom, or even outdoors. The adaptability of the game allows it to be customized to suit different age groups and skill levels, making it an inclusive activity that can engage all children. In my occupational therapy sessions, I have a different theme each week and use an obstacle course to search and find hidden themed objects – It's a lot of fun!

To set up the Hidden Object Concentration Game, you'll need common household items such as small toys, utensils, or everyday objects that are safe for children to handle. Begin by selecting a room or area where the game will take place. Hide these objects in various locations, ensuring that some are easy to find while others are more challenging. This variation in difficulty keeps the game interesting and helps children gradually improve their concentration skills. Once the objects are hidden, create a checklist of the items for your child to find. This checklist can include pictures or names of the objects, depending on your child's reading level.

For example, you might hide a small toy car under a cushion, a spoon on a bookshelf, and a sock behind a curtain. Write or draw these items on a piece of paper, and provide your child with the checklist. As they search for each item, they will need to focus their attention, remember the objects on the list, and use their problem-solving skills to find them. This process helps to enhance their attention span and develop their ability to stay on task.

To keep the game engaging, consider introducing different versions. You can add a timer to increase the challenge, encouraging your child to find all the objects within a set time frame. This adds an element of urgency and excitement, making the game more dynamic. Themed hunts are another way to maintain interest. For instance, during the holidays, you might hide holiday-themed objects like ornaments or small decorations. In the fall, you could use items related to autumn, such as leaves or mini pumpkins. Changing the theme periodically keeps the game fresh and exciting for your child.

The game can also be adapted to different rooms or outdoor spaces. Playing in a new environment introduces a novel challenge and prevents the game from becoming monotonous. For instance, an outdoor version might involve hiding objects in the backyard or a local park. This variation not only keeps the game exciting but also encourages children to explore and interact with different environments.

Parental involvement is key to the success of the Hidden Object Concentration Game. Participating in the game with your child can turn it into a collaborative activity that strengthens your bond. Offer guidance and support without taking over the search, allowing your child to experience the satisfaction of finding the objects independently. Observing your child's performance can provide valuable insights into their focus and attention levels. Notice if they become more efficient at finding objects over time and if their ability to stay on task improves. Providing positive feedback and celebrating their successes, no matter how small reinforces their efforts and builds their confidence.

REFLECTION SECTION: TRACKING PROGRESS

Create a simple chart to track your child's progress. List the objects they need to find and note how long it takes them to complete the search each time you play. Over a few weeks, compare the times to see if there is an improvement. Use this chart to discuss with your child how they feel about their progress and what strategies they found helpful. This reflective practice not only enhances their self-awareness but also reinforces the skills they are developing through the game.

The Hidden Object Concentration Game is a versatile and engaging way to help your child improve their focus and attention span. By incorporating different versions and settings, you can keep the activity fresh and exciting, ensuring that your child remains engaged and motivated. Please see The Hidden Object Concentration Game worksheet at the end of this chapter or print using the QR code at the beginning of the book.

2.2 TIME-BOUND TASK CHALLENGES

Time management is a crucial skill for children, helping them to improve focus and efficiency in their daily tasks. One effective way to teach this skill is through time-bound tasks. These tasks involve working within a set time frame, which can help children develop a sense of time awareness. By understanding how long certain activities take, children can learn to plan their time better and stay on track. This approach not only enhances their ability to concentrate but also instills a sense of responsibility and accomplishment.

Designing time-bound challenges can be simple and fun. Start with everyday household chores, such as tidying up a room within 10 minutes. Set a timer and encourage your child to see how much they can accomplish within that period. This not only makes the task more engaging but also helps them develop a sense of urgency and focus. Homework assignments can also be broken into timed segments. For instance, set a 20-minute timer for completing math problems, followed by a 5-minute break, and then another timed session for reading or writing tasks. This method helps children stay focused and prevents overwhelm by breaking tasks into manageable chunks.

Incorporating fun activities like puzzles and games with a timer can also be highly effective. Children love challenges, and adding a time element makes the activity more exciting. For example, set a timer for a jigsaw puzzle and see how much of it they can complete in 15 minutes. Alternatively, timed board games or digital apps that require quick thinking and decision-making can also be beneficial. These activities not only improve time management but also enhance cognitive skills and strategic thinking.

Tracking progress in these time-bound tasks is essential to help children see their improvement and stay motivated. Use charts and stickers to mark completed tasks. For instance, create a weekly chart where your child can add a sticker each time they complete a timed task. Visual representations of their progress can be highly motivating. Encourage self-assessment and reflection by discussing how they felt during the task and what strategies they used to stay focused. This reflection helps them become more aware of their abilities and areas for improvement.

Setting incremental goals and celebrating achievements is another effective way to keep children motivated. Start with simple tasks and gradually increase the difficulty level as your child becomes more comfortable with the concept of timed tasks. For example, if they can tidy up their room in 10 minutes, challenge them to do it in 8 minutes the next time. Similarly, if they can complete a puzzle in 20 minutes, try reducing the time to 18 minutes. Introducing multi-step tasks to complete within a time limit can also help develop their ability to plan and execute tasks efficiently. For instance, set a 30-minute timer for a series of tasks like completing a worksheet, reading a chapter, and organizing their desk.

Adjusting the difficulty levels based on your child's ability is crucial to ensure that the tasks remain challenging but achievable. Gradually decreasing the allotted time for tasks can push them to work more efficiently. On the other hand, increasing the complexity of the tasks can keep them engaged and help develop higher-order thinking skills. For example, a simple chore like setting the table can be turned into a complex task by adding elements like arranging the utensils in a specific order or creating a centerpiece.

Parental involvement in these time-bound tasks is vital. Participate in the challenges by setting your own timed tasks and working alongside your child. This not only makes the activity more enjoyable but also provides an opportunity for bonding and mutual support. Offer positive feedback and celebrate their successes, no matter how small. Observing your child's progress and providing encouragement can significantly impact their motivation and self-confidence.

VISUAL AID: TIME-BOUND TASK CHART

Create a simple weekly chart with columns for each day and rows for different tasks. Include sections for the task name, time allocated, and a space for stickers or checkmarks. This chart can help your child visualize their progress and stay motivated to complete their tasks within the given time frame.

Time-bound task challenges are a practical and engaging way to teach children time management. By incorporating everyday chores, homework assignments, and fun activities into timed sessions, you can help your child develop better focus, efficiency, and a sense of responsibility. Tracking progress, setting incremental goals, and adjusting difficulty levels ensure that the tasks remain challenging and rewarding.

2.3 FOCUSED BREATHING EXERCISES

Breathing exercises are a powerful tool for enhancing concentration and reducing stress. The simple act of controlled breathing can have profound effects on the nervous system, helping to calm the mind and body. When children practice focused breathing, they improve their mental focus, allowing them to stay attentive and engaged in their tasks. The connection between breathing and mental focus is well-documented; deep, rhythmic breathing sends signals to the brain that promote relaxation and concentration. Controlled breathing activates the parasympathetic nervous system, which counteracts the stress response and creates a sense of calm. This calming effect is particularly beneficial for children who struggle with anxiety or have difficulty staying focused.

One easy-to-follow breathing exercise is Balloon Breathing. This technique involves imagining inflating a balloon with each inhale. Ask your child to take a deep breath in, filling their lungs as if they are blowing up a balloon, then slowly exhale, releasing the air. This visualization helps them focus on their breath and makes the exercise more engaging. Another simple method is Counting Breaths. Have your child count each breath they take, inhaling and exhaling slowly while counting up to a certain number, such as ten. This counting helps maintain focus and can be particularly useful during moments of distraction or stress.

Box Breathing is another effective technique that involves inhaling, holding the breath, exhaling, and pausing for equal counts. To practice Box Breathing, instruct your child to inhale deeply for a count of four, hold the breath for another count of four, exhale slowly for a count of four, and then pause for a final count of four before repeating the cycle. This structured pattern of breathing helps regulate the nervous system and promotes a state of calm focus. The equal counts make it easy to remember and practice, even in situations where your child might feel anxious or overwhelmed.

Incorporating breathing exercises into your child's daily routine can significantly enhance their concentration and reduce stress. Starting the day with a brief breathing exercise sets a positive tone. Encourage your child to spend a few minutes practicing Balloon Breathing or Box Breathing before heading to school. This can help them feel more centered and ready to face the day's challenges. Using breathing techniques before homework or tests can also be beneficial. Taking a few deep breaths can calm the mind and improve focus, making it easier for your child to concentrate on their work. Practicing breathing before bedtime can promote better sleep. A calm, relaxed state helps children fall asleep more easily and enjoy a restful night.

Your support is crucial in helping your child practice these breathing exercises. Modeling the exercises for your child can be highly effective. Practice the techniques together, showing them how to inhale deeply, hold their breath, and exhale slowly. Creating a calm environment for practice is also important. Choose a quiet, comfortable space where your child can focus on their breath without distractions. Encourage consistency and regular practice by integrating these exercises into daily routines. The more your child practices, the more natural and effective these techniques will become.

For instance, you might start each morning with a few minutes of Box Breathing, practice Counting Breaths before homework sessions, and end the day with Balloon Breathing before bedtime. Observing your child's responses to these exercises can provide valuable insights. Notice any changes in their ability to concentrate, their stress levels, and their overall mood. Provide positive feedback and celebrate their efforts, reinforcing the benefits of regular practice.

By integrating focused breathing exercises into your child's routine, you can help them develop a valuable tool for enhancing concentration and reducing stress. These simple techniques are easy to learn and practice, making them an accessible and effective way to support your child's mental and emotional well-being. Your involvement and support play a crucial role in encouraging regular practice and helping your child reap the full benefits of these exercises.

2.4 CREATING A DISTRACTION-FREE HOMEWORK ZONE

Creating a dedicated homework space for your child is important for promoting focus and concentration. A distraction-free area reduces interruptions and helps your child stay on task. It also creates a routine, signaling the brain that it's time to work. When a child has a specific place to do their homework, it becomes easier for them to switch into "work mode," making the completion of tasks smoother and more efficient.

To set up an ideal homework zone, start by choosing a quiet, well-lit area in your home. This could be a corner of their bedroom, a spot in the living room, or even a small nook in the kitchen. The key is to find a place where your child can work without constant disruptions. Ensure that the workspace is organized and clutter-free. A tidy environment reduces distractions and helps your child find the materials they need quickly. Provide necessary supplies within easy reach, such as pencils, erasers, paper, and any other tools they regularly use for their homework. This setup minimizes the need to get up and search for items, which can break their concentration.

Minimizing distractions is another essential aspect of creating an effective homework zone. Limit access to electronic devices that are not needed for homework. If your child needs a computer or tablet for their assignments, ensure that it's used strictly for school-related tasks. Using noise-canceling headphones or white noise machines can help block out background noise, making it easier for your child to focus. Establish clear rules for siblings and pets during homework time. Let everyone in the household know that this is a quiet period, and interruptions should be kept to a minimum.

Personalizing the homework zone can make it more inviting and motivating for your child. Allow them to decorate the area with personal items, such as photos, drawings, or favorite quotes. This makes the space feel like their own and can increase their willingness to spend time there. Using motivational posters and goal charts can also be effective. Visual reminders of their goals and achievements can provide an extra boost of motivation. Incorporating comfortable seating and proper ergonomics is important for maintaining focus and preventing fatigue. Ensure that the chair and desk are at the right height for your child, and consider adding a cushion or footrest if needed.

Creating a distraction-free homework zone is a key step in helping your child develop better focus and concentration. By providing a quiet, organized, and personalized space, you can support their ability to complete tasks efficiently and with greater ease. This dedicated area not only enhances their current academic performance but also instills habits that will benefit them in the long run.

In the next chapter, we will explore strategies and activities to improve instruction-following skills, helping your child become more independent and successful in their daily tasks.

Activity Worksheet

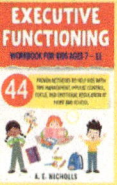

Chapter 2 — Focus & Concentration

Activity: The Hidden Object Concentration Game

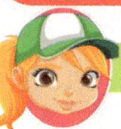

Household Items Checklist:
- Spoon
- Toy Car
- Book
- Block
- Pencil
- Cup
- Ball
- Key
- Shoe
- Hat
- Coin

Draw a Map:
- Draw the locations where you hid or found the items below:

Reflection Section:

Date	Objects to Find	Time Taken (mins)	Challenges Faced	Strategies Used	Reflections/ Feelings	Improvement Noted
09/22	Spoon, Car, Ball	10	Distracted by noise	Focused on one area	Felt frustrated at first	Yes/No

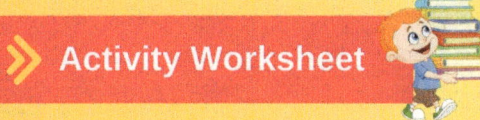 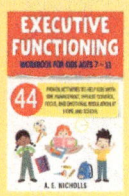

Activity Worksheet

Chapter 2 — **Focus & Concentration**

 **Activity:** Time-Bound Task Challenges

Weekly Task Chart:

Day	Task	Time Allotted	Sticker
Monday	Example: Tidy up room	10 minutes	
Tuesday			
Wednesday			
Thursday			
Friday			
Saturday			
Sunday			

Reflection section

- What strategies helped you complete your tasks faster this week?

- Were there any tasks that took longer than expected? Why?

- How do you feel about your progress this week?

>> Activity Worksheet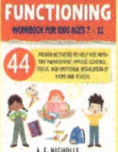

Chapter 2 — Focus & Concentration

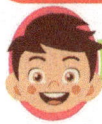 **Activity:** Focused Breathing Exercises

What You Need:

- Take a deep breath in through your nose for 4 seconds.
- Hold your breath for 4 seconds.
- Slowly breathe out through your mouth for 4 seconds.
- Color in one of the circles around the bear after each deep breath.
- Repeat until all five circles are colored in.

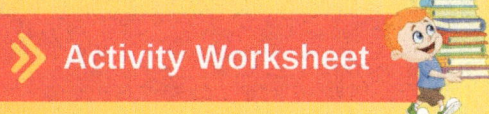 **Activity Worksheet**

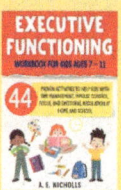

Chapter 2 — Focus & Concentration

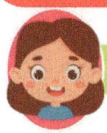 **Activity:** Creating a Distraction-Free Homework Zone

Checklist: Set Up Your Distraction-Free Zone

1. Comfortable Desk and Chair

○ My chair is comfortable and helps me sit up straight.

○ My desk is the right height for writing or using a computer.

2. Adequate Lighting

○ My space gets natural light from a window.

○ I have a desk lamp or overhead light that isn't too bright or too dim.

3. Organized Bookshelf

○ I've placed my bookshelf near my desk for easy access to books and supplies.

○ My bookshelf is organized so everything is easy to find.

4. Clutter-Free Workspace

○ My desk is clear of unnecessary items like toys or gadgets.

○ Only the things I need for homework are on my desk.

5. Quiet Environment

○ My homework space is away from noisy areas like the TV or kitchen.

○ I've turned off or silenced any electronics that might distract me.

6. Personal Touches

○ I've added something small to my workspace that makes me happy, like a plant or photo.

○ I made sure not to put too many decorations to avoid distractions.

3

IMPROVING INSTRUCTION-FOLLOWING SKILLS

"Children need models rather than critics."

— JOSEPH JOUBERT

Consider the morning routine of seven-year-old Ben. Each day, he seems to struggle with remembering and completing basic tasks like brushing his teeth, getting dressed, and packing his school bag. His mom, Jessica, often finds herself repeating instructions multiple times, only to end up doing half the tasks for him. This situation can be frustrating for both Ben and Jessica, leading to stressful mornings. The solution to this common challenge lies in improving Ben's ability to follow instructions and develop a sense of responsibility. One effective tool to achieve this is the use of chore charts.

3.1 STEP-BY-STEP CHORE CHARTS

Chore charts are invaluable in teaching children responsibility and the ability to follow instructions. They help children understand and remember their daily tasks by providing a clear, visual representation of what needs to be done. When children see their tasks laid out in a chart, it becomes easier for them to follow through without constant reminders. This visual aid also tracks progress and completion, offering a sense of achievement as tasks are marked off. By using chore charts, children learn to take ownership of their responsibilities, fostering independence and accountability. This practice not only benefits their daily routines but also builds a foundation for future organizational skills.

Creating an effective chore chart involves several key elements. First, use clear and simple language for each task. This ensures that your child knows exactly what is expected of them. For children who struggle to read, incorporating visual aids like pictures can be particularly helpful. For example, use an image of a toothbrush next to the task "Brush Teeth" or a picture of a bed next to "Make Bed." These visual cues make the chart accessible and engaging for children who are not yet proficient readers. Additionally, break down larger chores into smaller, manageable steps. Instead of listing "Clean Room" as one task, break it down into "Pick Up Toys," "Put Clothes in Hamper," and "Make Bed." This approach makes the tasks feel less overwhelming and more achievable.

To implement the chore chart system effectively, start by setting a consistent time each day to review the chart with your child. This could be in the morning before school or in the evening before bed. Reviewing the chart together helps reinforce the routine and allows you to provide any necessary guidance. Encourage your child to mark off completed tasks themselves. This act of marking off tasks gives them a sense of control and accomplishment. To keep them motivated, offer rewards or incentives for completing all their chores. These can be simple, such as a sticker for each completed task or extra playtime at the end of the week. Rewards help reinforce the positive behavior of following instructions and completing tasks.

Examples of chore charts can vary based on the age and needs of the child. For younger children, a morning routine chart might include tasks like "Brush Teeth," "Make Bed," and "Get Dressed." Each task can be accompanied by a picture to make it more engaging. A weekly chore chart for slightly older children could include tasks such as "Take Out Trash," "Feed Pets," and "Vacuum Room." This chart can help them keep track of their responsibilities throughout the week. For children involved in various activities, a responsibility chart might include "Complete Homework," "Attend Extracurricular Activities," and "Family Time." This type of chart helps balance schoolwork, hobbies, and family commitments.

VISUAL AID: SAMPLE CHORE CHART TEMPLATE

Create a simple template for a chore chart that includes columns for the day of the week, tasks, and a space for checkmarks or stickers. This template can be customized based on your child's specific responsibilities and age.

By introducing chore charts, you give your child a practical tool to improve their instruction-following skills. This method not only makes daily routines smoother but also instills a sense of responsibility and independence. Your involvement in creating and maintaining the chore chart system is essential. By working together, you can help your child develop the skills they need to be successful and organized in their daily life.

3.2 SIMON SAYS WITH A TWIST

The classic game of "Simon Says" is a childhood favorite that does much more than entertain. It's a simple game where one person takes on the role of Simon and gives commands that others must follow, but only if the command begins with "Simon says." This game is excellent for enhancing listening skills and attention to detail. Children must listen carefully to follow directions accurately, learning to differentiate between commands that require action and those that do not. The interactive nature of the game makes learning fun, allowing children to practice following instructions in an engaging way.

To make "Simon Says" more challenging and educational, you can introduce multi-step instructions. For example, "Simon says, jump three times and then touch your toes" combines physical actions that require children to remember and execute multiple steps. Conditional instructions add another layer of complexity. You might say, "Simon says, if you're wearing blue, hop on one foot." This requires children to process the condition and then decide if it applies to them, enhancing their cognitive flexibility. Incorporating physical and cognitive tasks can make the game even more enriching. For instance, "Simon says, spell your name while clapping" combines spelling with a physical activity, promoting both mental and physical coordination.

Playing "Simon Says" in groups offers additional benefits for social skills development. Group play encourages teamwork and cooperation as children learn to wait for their turn and follow group dynamics. It also promotes healthy competition and sportsmanship. Children who wait patiently for their turn and cheer for their peers develop a sense of camaraderie and mutual respect. These social interactions are crucial for building relationships and learning to work together, skills that are valuable both in and out of the classroom.

Parental participation can elevate the learning experience in "Simon Says." Playing the game during family time not only bonds the family but also provides an opportunity for parents to observe and reinforce their child's ability to follow instructions. Use the game as a fun break during homework or study sessions to refresh your child's mind while still practicing important skills. As you play, observe how your child follows instructions and provide positive feedback. Praise their efforts and successes, reinforcing the importance of listening and following directions accurately. This positive reinforcement encourages them to continue applying these skills in other areas of their life.

Imagine a typical game where you say, "Simon says, stand on one leg and count to five." Your child must listen, process the command, and execute it accurately. If you follow with, "Touch your head," without the "Simon says" prefix, they must resist the urge to follow the command. This practice sharpens their listening skills and impulse control, essential components of executive functioning. The game's simplicity allows for endless variations, keeping it fresh and challenging each time you play.

In the next sub-chapter, we will explore how following recipes can further enhance your child's ability to follow multi-step instructions, combining practical skills with fun and interactive learning.

3.3 RECIPE FOLLOWING FOR KIDS

Cooking is a fantastic way to teach children how to follow multi-step instructions while combining reading, measuring, and sequencing skills. When your child follows a recipe, they engage in a hands-on learning experience that requires them to read instructions, measure ingredients accurately, and follow a specific sequence of steps. This process not only reinforces their ability to follow directions but also builds their confidence and independence in the kitchen. Cooking allows children to see the tangible results of their efforts, giving them a sense of accomplishment and pride in their creations.

Choosing kid-friendly recipes is key to ensuring that the cooking experience is both enjoyable and safe. Start with easy-to-follow recipes that have clear, simple steps. Opt for recipes that use basic ingredients and kitchen tools to minimize complexity. For younger children, select recipes that require minimal cooking or supervision, such as no-bake treats or simple sandwiches. For instance, making a fruit salad involves washing, cutting, and mixing fruits—tasks that are straightforward and safe with proper supervision. Preparing a sandwich is another excellent activity that teaches layering ingredients in a specific order, reinforcing the concept of following steps. Baking cookies can be a bit more complex, but it is highly rewarding. Measuring ingredients, mixing dough, and using cookie cutters provide a comprehensive learning experience while being fun and interactive.

When engaging children in cooking activities, safety and supervision are paramount. Always supervise your child when they are using sharp tools or handling hot surfaces. Teach them essential kitchen safety rules, such as washing hands before handling food, keeping the cooking area clean, and wiping up spills immediately to prevent accidents. Encourage your child to ask for help when needed, especially with tasks that involve knives, hot stoves, or ovens. For example, if your child is cutting fruit for a salad, guide their hands and show them the proper way to hold and use a knife. When baking cookies, handle the oven duties yourself while explaining the process to your child.

Consider the case of preparing a fruit salad. Start by gathering a variety of fruits like apples, bananas, and berries. Have your child wash the fruits thoroughly. This simple step teaches them the importance of hygiene in cooking. Next, guide them through cutting the fruits into bite-sized pieces. Depending on their age and skill level, you can supervise closely or let them handle the cutting with a safe, child-friendly knife. Once all the fruits are cut, let your child mix them in a large bowl. This activity involves following a sequence of steps, from washing to cutting to mixing, reinforcing their ability to follow multi-step instructions.

Another example is making a sandwich. Gather all the ingredients, such as bread, cheese, lettuce, and deli meat. Lay them out in the order they will be used. Guide your child through layering the ingredients, starting with spreading a condiment on the bread, adding the cheese and meat, and finally topping it with lettuce before closing the sandwich. This activity not only teaches them to follow a sequence but also allows for creativity in choosing and arranging ingredients.

Baking cookies provides a more complex yet highly rewarding cooking experience. Begin by having your child measure the ingredients. Show them how to level off dry ingredients like flour and sugar to ensure accuracy. Let them crack the eggs into a separate bowl to avoid shells in the dough. As they mix the ingredients, explain the importance of following the recipe's order to achieve the best results. Using cookie cutters to shape the dough adds an element of fun and creativity. Throughout the process, supervise closely, especially when using the oven.

Incorporating these cooking activities into your routine not only helps your child develop executive functioning skills but also provides valuable bonding time. They learn to follow instructions, work independently, and take pride in their accomplishments. By choosing simple, safe recipes and providing appropriate supervision and guidance, you can create a positive, educational experience in the kitchen.

3.4 BUILDING MODELS WITH INSTRUCTIONS

Building models is a great activity for developing a range of skills in children. Engaging in model building enhances spatial awareness and fine motor skills as children manipulate small parts and pieces to create a larger structure. This hands-on activity requires them to visualize how different components fit together, improving their ability to understand and navigate space. Also, building models teaches patience and attention to detail. Children must follow precise steps and focus on each part of the process, which cultivates a sense of discipline and thoroughness. The sense of accomplishment upon completing a model is significant. Seeing the finished product reinforces the value of perseverance and effort, boosting their confidence and self-esteem.

Selecting the right type of model for your child is essential to ensure that the activity is both challenging and enjoyable. For younger children, simple block structures are an excellent starting point. These can include basic building blocks or larger, interlocking pieces that are easy to handle. As children grow older and their skills improve, pre-cut cardboard or plastic models become more appropriate. These models often come with pieces that need to be assembled in a specific order, requiring more detailed attention and fine motor coordination. For older children who seek a more complex challenge, detailed kits with multiple parts are ideal. These kits often include small, intricate pieces and may involve various stages of assembly, providing a more rewarding and immersive experience.

Following instruction manuals is a fundamental part of the model-building process. Encourage your child to read through all the instructions before starting. This helps them understand the overall scope of the project and anticipate the steps involved. Breaking down the steps into smaller tasks makes the process more manageable. For instance, focus on completing one section of the model before moving on to the next. This approach prevents overwhelm and keeps the child engaged. Visual aids and diagrams are helpful for understanding complex steps. Instruction manuals often include detailed illustrations that show how pieces fit together. Encourage your child to refer to these diagrams frequently, as they provide a clear guide to assembly.

Parental support and engagement play a significant role in making model building a successful and enjoyable activity. Participate in the project as a team activity. Working together not only makes the process more fun but also provides an opportunity for bonding. Offer guidance and assistance without taking over. Allow your child to take the lead and make decisions, stepping in only when they need help. This fosters independence and problem-solving skills. Celebrate the completion of each step and the final model. Acknowledge the effort and dedication your child has put into the project. This positive reinforcement encourages them to tackle more complex models in the future.

Imagine working on a detailed plastic model of a car with your child. Start by laying out all the pieces and reviewing the instruction manual together. Discuss the steps involved and identify any parts that might be challenging. As you progress, take breaks to review your work and ensure each piece is correctly placed. This not only reinforces the importance of following instructions but also provides an opportunity to correct any mistakes before moving on. By the time the model is complete, your child will have gained valuable skills in spatial awareness, patience, and attention to detail, along with the pride of seeing their hard work come to fruition.

In summary, building models is a multi-layered activity that supports the development of essential skills in children. By selecting age-appropriate models, encouraging thorough reading of instructions, and providing supportive engagement, you can help your child enhance their spatial awareness, fine motor skills, patience, and attention to detail. These skills are invaluable for their academic and personal growth, setting a strong foundation for future success.

In the next chapter, we will explore how emotional regulation techniques can further support your child's development, providing them with tools to manage their emotions effectively in different situations.

Activity Worksheet

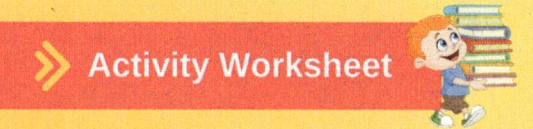

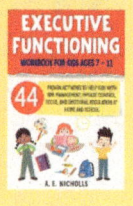

Chapter 3 — Following Instructions

Activity: Step-by-Step Chore Charts

Weekly Task Chart:

Chores	Monday	Tuesday	Wednesday	Thursday	Friday	Saturday	Sunday
Brush Teeth							
Make Bed							
Pick Up Toys							
Put Clothes in Hamper							
Help Set the Table							
Family Time							
Complete Homework							
Read for 20 Minutes							

Reflection Corner for Kids:

1. Which chore was your favorite to do this week?
2. Was there a chore you found hard? How can we make it easier?
3. What chore made you feel proud?
4. Is there a new chore you'd like to learn next week?

Activity Worksheet

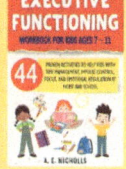

Chapter 3 — Following Instructions

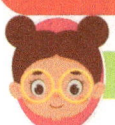

Activity: Simon Says with a Twist

Instructions:

1. One player will act as Simon and give multi-step commands.
2. The commands can be anything Simon says, like "touch your nose, clap three times, and spin around."
3. Players must follow each step of the command in order, but only if Simon starts with "Simon says." If Simon doesn't say "Simon says," the players should not follow the command.
4. If a player follows a command without "Simon says," they are out for that round.
5. Simon can issue multiple steps in one command, increasing the challenge!

Example of a command:

- Simon says touch your toes, jump twice, and say your name.

Commands List:

1. _____
2. _____
3. _____
4. _____
5. _____
6. _____
7. _____
8. _____
9. _____
10. _____

Reflection:

- What strategies helped you remember the commands?
_____
_____

>> **Activity Worksheet**

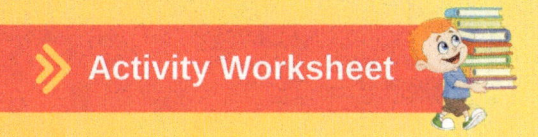

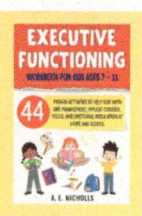

Chapter 3 — **Following Instructions**

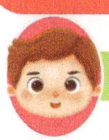

Activity: Recipe Following for Kids

- **Recipe Name :** _____

Ingredients:

- (✓ Check off each ingredient as you gather them)
  - ○ ------------------------------
  - ○ ------------------------------
  - ○ ------------------------------
  - ○ ------------------------------
  - ○ ------------------------------
  - ○ ------------------------------
  - ○ ------------------------------
  - ○ ------------------------------
  - ○ ------------------------------

Steps:

- (✓ Check off each step as you complete it)
  - ○ ------------------------------
  - ○ ------------------------------
  - ○ ------------------------------
  - ○ ------------------------------
  - ○ ------------------------------
  - ○ ------------------------------
  - ○ ------------------------------
  - ○ ------------------------------
  - ○ ------------------------------

My Notes:

- (Write down your adjustments, tips, or thoughts on the recipe)

Reflection:

- What was the most challenging part of following this recipe?

- What did you enjoy the most about this recipe?

Activity Worksheet

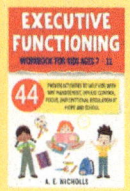

Chapter 3 — Following Instructions

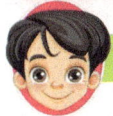

Activity: Building Models with Instructions

Instructions:
- Write each step of your model-building process in the lines below
- Use the space on the right for drawings or diagrams to help explain each step visually.

Step	Written Instructions	Drawing/Diagram (optional)
1.		
2.		
3.		
4.		
5.		
6.		
7.		
8.		
9.		
10.		

Reflection:
- How did writing instructions help you understand the building process better?

4

EMOTIONAL REGULATION TECHNIQUES

"One of the greatest gifts you can give your children is the ability to manage their emotions. It helps them navigate life's challenges with resilience and grace."

— DANIEL J. SIEGEL

One evening, ten-year-old Lily had a meltdown over a seemingly minor issue—her favorite shirt was still in the laundry. Her dad, Tom, felt helpless as he watched Lily's frustration escalate into tears and shouting. He wished he knew how to help her manage her emotions better. Emotional regulation is a critical skill for children, enabling them to handle stress, frustration, and other intense feelings in a healthy way. This chapter will explore practical techniques to help your child develop better emotional regulation skills, starting with the power of mindfulness.

4.1 MINDFULNESS FOR KIDS

Mindfulness is a practice that involves being present in the moment without judgment. It teaches children to focus on their current experience, whether it's their breath, a sound, or a physical sensation, without getting caught up in thoughts about the past or future. The benefits of mindfulness for children are substantial. It enhances focus, reduces stress, and improves emotional regulation. Practicing mindfulness helps children become more aware of their thoughts and feelings, giving them tools to manage their emotions more effectively.

This practice is suitable in different settings, including school, home, and social situations, making it a versatile tool for emotional development.

Introducing mindfulness to children can be simple and enjoyable. Mindful coloring is one effective activity. Provide your child with coloring sheets and encourage them to focus on staying within the lines and choosing colors mindfully. This activity not only promotes concentration but also provides a calming outlet for self-expression. Sensory awareness exercises are another great way to practice mindfulness. Ask your child to pay attention to the sounds, smells, and textures around them. For example, during a walk in the park, have them close their eyes and describe the sounds they hear or the feel of different leaves and stones. This activity helps children become more attuned to their environment and enhances their sensory perception.

A body scan is another simple yet powerful mindfulness exercise. Guide your child to notice different parts of their body and how they feel. Have them start at their toes and slowly move up to their head, paying attention to any sensations they experience. This practice helps children connect with their bodies and develop a greater awareness of physical and emotional states. It can be particularly useful before bedtime as it promotes relaxation and prepares the body for restful sleep.

Incorporating mindfulness into daily routines can make these practices a natural part of your child's life. Mindful eating is an excellent way to integrate mindfulness into mealtime. Encourage your child to focus on the taste, texture, and smell of their food. Have them take small bites and chew slowly, paying attention to each sensation. This practice not only enhances their enjoyment of food but also promotes healthier eating habits. Mindful walking is another way to practice mindfulness during everyday activities. Whether walking to school or taking a stroll in the park, encourage your child to pay attention to each step, the ground beneath their feet, and their surroundings. This practice helps them stay present and connected to their environment.

Mindful listening is a valuable exercise that can be practiced during conversations. Encourage your child to listen actively and attentively when someone is speaking without interrupting or thinking about their response. This practice improves communication skills and fosters empathy and understanding. It also helps children become more aware of their own thoughts and feelings during interactions, promoting better emotional regulation.

Your involvement in practicing mindfulness with your child is crucial for their success. Participate in mindfulness exercises together to model the behavior and show your support. Create a calm and quiet environment for practice, free from distractions and interruptions. This space can be as simple as a corner of a room with comfortable seating and soft lighting.

Encourage consistency by making mindfulness a regular part of the day. For example, start each morning with a brief mindfulness exercise or end the day with a body scan before bedtime. Consistent practice helps reinforce the benefits of mindfulness and makes it a habitual part of your child's routine.

By incorporating these mindfulness techniques into your child's daily life, you can help them develop valuable skills for managing their emotions. Mindfulness not only enhances focus and reduces stress but also provides a foundation for emotional well-being. Your support and participation make a significant difference in helping your child embrace and benefit from these practices.

4.2 THE CALM DOWN JAR ACTIVITY

The Calm Down Jar is a practical tool designed to help children manage their emotions. This visual aid captures their focus and provides a tangible method for calming down. When children shake the jar and watch the glitter slowly settle, it encourages them to take deep breaths and practice mindfulness. This simple yet effective tool helps them center their thoughts and emotions, making it easier to regain control during moments of distress. The Calm Down Jar offers a specific, hands-on way to cope with overwhelming feelings, giving children a sense of control over their emotional responses.

To create a Calm Down Jar, you will need a few basic materials. Start with a clear plastic or glass jar with a lid. The clarity of the jar is important as it allows children to see the glitter swirling and settling. Next, gather water, glitter glue, and food coloring. The glitter glue serves as the main ingredient that creates a mesmerizing effect when the jar is shaken. Food coloring adds a touch of color, making the jar more visually appealing. If you want to enhance the effect, you can also include small beads or sequins. These additional elements add variety and make the settling process even more engaging for the child.

Making a Calm Down Jar is a straightforward process. Begin by filling the jar with water, leaving some space at the top to allow for shaking. Next, add a generous amount of glitter glue to the water. The quantity of glitter glue will determine how long it takes for the glitter to settle, so you can adjust this based on how long you want the calming effect to last. After adding the glitter glue, include a few drops of food coloring to give the water a vibrant hue. Stir the mixture well to ensure the glitter glue and food coloring are evenly distributed. Once everything is mixed, seal the jar tightly to prevent any leaks. Give the jar a good shake to see the effect. The glitter should swirl around and gradually settle, creating a soothing visual display.

Using the Calm Down Jar effectively involves a few key steps. When your child is feeling upset or overwhelmed, encourage them to shake the jar and watch the glitter settle. This action serves as a distraction, redirecting their focus from their distress to the calming movement of the glitter. As they watch the glitter, guide them to take deep breaths. Inhale slowly through the nose, hold for a moment, and then exhale gently through the mouth. This combination of visual and breathing exercises helps to calm the nervous system and reduce emotional intensity. The Calm Down Jar can also serve as a signal for a quiet time or break. If your child is experiencing a meltdown, suggest using the jar as a cue to step away from the situation and take a moment to calm down.

REFLECTION SECTION: CREATING A CALM-DOWN ROUTINE

Consider setting up a dedicated space for your child to use their Calm Down Jar. This space can include comfortable seating, soft lighting, and other calming elements like stuffed animals or a favorite blanket. Encourage your child to use this space and their jar whenever they need to calm down. Establishing a routine where they use the jar and take deep breaths can make this practice more effective. Reflect with your child on how they feel before and after using the jar, discussing the benefits they notice in their ability to manage their emotions.

The Calm Down Jar is a versatile and engaging tool that provides children with a concrete method for managing their emotions. By incorporating this activity into their routine, you offer them a valuable resource for navigating emotional challenges. Your involvement in creating and using the Calm Down Jar reinforces its effectiveness, helping your child develop better emotional regulation skills. Please see the wonderful Calm Down Jar activity at the end of this chapter or print using the QR code in the introduction.

4.3 EMOTION IDENTIFICATION CARDS

Helping children recognize and name their emotions is a crucial part of emotional regulation. When children can understand and express their feelings, they are better equipped to handle them constructively. This skill reduces instances of emotional outbursts as children learn to identify what they are feeling before the emotion becomes overwhelming. Additionally, recognizing emotions promotes empathy and social skills. When children can name their own feelings, they become more attuned to the emotions of others, fostering healthier interactions and relationships.

Creating emotion identification cards is a simple yet powerful tool to help children develop this skill. Start with index cards or print templates that depict various emotions. Each card should include a picture or drawing representing the emotion, such as a smiling face for happiness or a frowning face for sadness. Alongside the image, write the name of the emotion and a brief description. For example, a card with a picture of an angry face might include the word "Angry" and a description like "Feeling upset and frustrated." These cards serve as visual aids that make it easier for children to understand and label their emotions.

Incorporating emotion identification cards into daily routines can be both practical and beneficial. Begin each day with a morning check-in, where your child picks a card that represents how they feel. This practice helps them start the day with self-awareness and opens the door for discussions about their emotions. During reflection time, use the cards to talk about the emotions experienced throughout the day. Ask your child to pick cards that match their feelings during different events, helping them process and understand their emotional responses. When conflicts arise, these cards can be helpful for problem-solving. Encourage your child to identify the emotions involved in the conflict and discuss ways to address them constructively.

Interactive activities with emotion identification cards can make learning about emotions fun and engaging. One such activity is Emotion Charades. In this game, a child picks a card and acts out the emotion without speaking while others guess the emotion being portrayed. This activity not only reinforces the recognition of emotions but also enhances non-verbal communication skills. Emotion Stories is another engaging activity. Have your child draw a card and create a story based on that emotion. For example, if they pick a card that says "Happy," they might tell a story about a joyful day at the park. This activity encourages creativity and helps children explore different emotional scenarios.

Emotion Match is an additional interactive game that helps children connect emotions with situations. Create a set of cards with various situations, such as "Losing a toy" or "Winning a game," and have your child match these situation cards with the corresponding emotion cards. This game not only reinforces the understanding of emotions but also helps children learn to anticipate and recognize emotional responses in different contexts.

VISUAL AID: EMOTION IDENTIFICATION CARD TEMPLATE

To help you get started, here is a simple template for creating emotion identification cards. Draw or print a picture of the emotion in the top half of the card. Below the picture, write the name of the emotion, followed by a brief description. For instance, for "Sad," you might include a picture of a tearful face, the word "Sad," and a description like "Feeling unhappy and wanting to cry."

Using emotion identification cards regularly can significantly enhance your child's ability to recognize and manage their emotions. By making these cards a part of your daily routine and incorporating them into interactive activities, you provide your child with valuable tools for emotional regulation. Your involvement in creating and using these cards is essential. By working together, you can help your child navigate their emotions more effectively, fostering a sense of empathy and improving their social skills.

4.4 BREATHING TECHNIQUES FOR EMOTIONAL CONTROL

Controlled breathing is a powerful tool for emotional regulation. It calms the nervous system, reduces stress, and enhances focus. By managing strong emotions and impulses, children can handle difficult situations more effectively. Deep, rhythmic breathing sends calming signals to the brain, helping to shift from a state of stress to one of relaxation. This physiological change makes it easier to manage emotions and maintain concentration, providing children with a simple yet effective way to improve their emotional health.

Several easy-to-follow breathing exercises can be particularly beneficial for children. One such exercise is Bubble Breathing. Ask your child to imagine they are blowing bubbles. Encourage them to take a deep breath in, then exhale slowly as if they are gently blowing a bubble. This visualization makes the exercise engaging and fun, helping children focus on their breath and calm down. Another technique is Flower Breath. Have your child pretend to smell a flower. Instruct them to inhale deeply through their nose, imagining the sweet scent of a flower, and then exhale slowly through their mouth. This exercise combines deep breathing with a pleasant visualization, making it both calming and enjoyable.

The 4-7-8 Breathing technique is another effective method that is similar to box breathing in Chapter 2. Guide your child to inhale through their nose for a count of four, hold their breath for a count of seven, and then exhale through their mouth for a count of eight. This structured pattern helps regulate the breath and calm the mind, making it a useful tool for managing stress and anxiety. Practicing these techniques regularly can help children develop better control over their emotions, improving their overall well-being.

Incorporating breathing exercises into daily routines can make them a natural part of your child's life. Encourage your child to practice these techniques before starting homework or schoolwork. Taking a few deep breaths can help clear their mind and prepare them for focused activity. During transitions between activities, such as moving from playtime to mealtime, suggest a quick breathing exercise to help them switch gears smoothly. Integrating these practices into bedtime routines can also promote relaxation and better sleep. A few minutes of deep breathing before bed can help your child unwind and prepare for a restful night.

Like the other activities, your guidance and support are essential in helping your child practice these breathing techniques. Model the exercises for your child, demonstrating how to take deep, slow breaths. Creating a calm environment for practice can enhance the effectiveness of these exercises. Choose a quiet, comfortable space where your child can focus on their breath without distractions. Encourage regular practice by making these exercises a consistent part of their daily routine. Positive reinforcement is also important. Praise your child for their efforts and the improvements they make, reinforcing the value of these practices.

Imagine your child practicing Bubble Breathing before a challenging task. They take a deep breath in, then slowly exhale as if blowing a bubble. This simple action helps them calm down and focus, making it easier to handle the task at hand. Or consider them using Flower Breath during a moment of frustration. By imagining the scent of a flower and taking deep breaths, they can shift from a state of stress to one of calm, managing their emotions more effectively.

Incorporating these breathing techniques into your child's routine can provide them with valuable tools for emotional regulation. Your involvement and support make a significant difference in their ability to practice and benefit from these exercises. By helping your child develop these skills, you contribute to their emotional health and resilience, preparing them to handle life's challenges with greater ease.

In this chapter, we have explored various techniques to help children develop emotional regulation skills. From mindfulness exercises and calm-down jars to emotion identification cards and controlled breathing techniques, these tools provide practical ways to support your child's emotional development. By integrating these practices into daily routines, you can help your child build a strong foundation for emotional well-being. Next, we will delve into strategies for improving time management skills, offering practical activities to help your child stay organized and focused.

Activity Worksheet

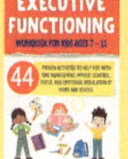

Chapter 3 — Following Instructions

Activity: Mindfulness for Kids

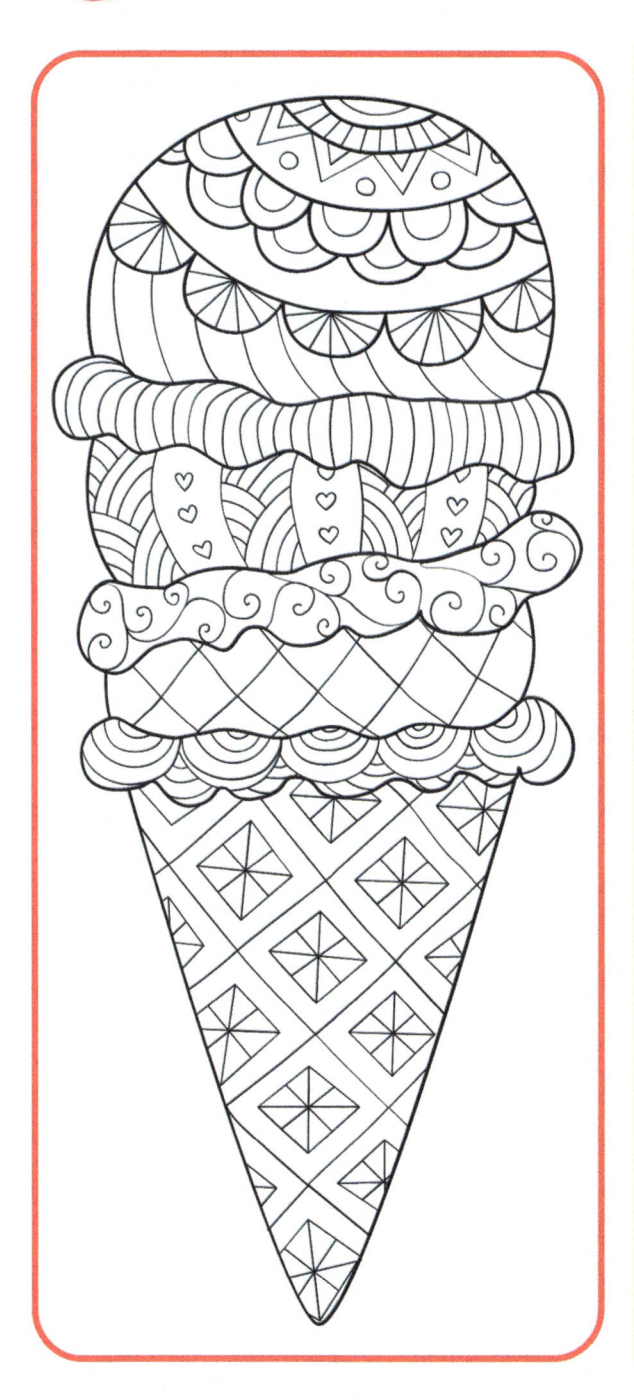

1. Color Together
   - ○ Join in
   - ○ Be present
2. Make a Calm Space
   - ○ Quiet spot
   - ○ Comfortable
   - ○ Soft light
3. Make It a Routine
   - ○ Daily practice
   - ○ Start small
4. Stay Mindful While Coloring
   - ○ Focus on colors
   - ○ Focus on strokes
   - ○ Deep breaths
   - ○ Refocus
5. Reflect After Coloring
   - ○ Talk about feelings
   - ○ Praise their focus
   - ○ Celebrate

Activity Worksheet

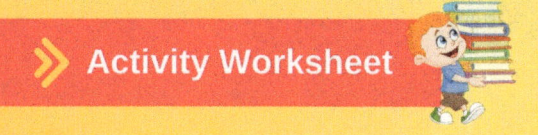

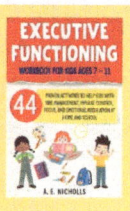

Chapter 4 — Emotional Regulation

Activity: The Calm Down Jar Activity

What You Need:

- (✓ Check off each material as you gather them)
  - [ ] A clear plastic or glass jar with a lid
  - [ ] Warm water
  - [ ] Glitter glue or clear glue
  - [ ] Fine glitter (various colors)
  - [ ] Food coloring (optional)
  - [ ] Super glue or hot glue (to seal the lid)

Instructions:

- (✓ Check off each step as you complete it)
  - [ ] Fill the jar about 3/4 full with warm water.
  - [ ] Add about 1-2 tablespoons of glitter glue (or clear glue). Stir until it's fully mixed.
  - [ ] Add a few drops of food coloring if you want to give the water a different color. Stir to mix.
  - [ ] Sprinkle a tablespoon of fine glitter into the jar. Feel free to use multiple colors!
  - [ ] Stir well to make sure everything is blended.
  - [ ] Add more water to the jar until it's almost full, leaving a small gap at the top.
  - [ ] Seal the lid tightly using super glue or hot glue so it doesn't leak.
  - [ ] Shake your jar and watch the glitter swirl around!

Draw Your Finished Calm Down Jar:

- (Use this space to draw what your Calm Down Jar looks like!)

Reflection:

- When do you think using your Calm Down Jar would be most helpful?

Activity Worksheet

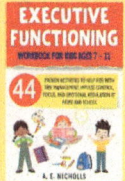

Chapter 4: Emotional Regulation

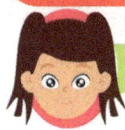

Activity: Emotion Identification Cards

Emotion Name:

"I feel this way when..."
When I feel this way, I can..."

Emotion prompt list

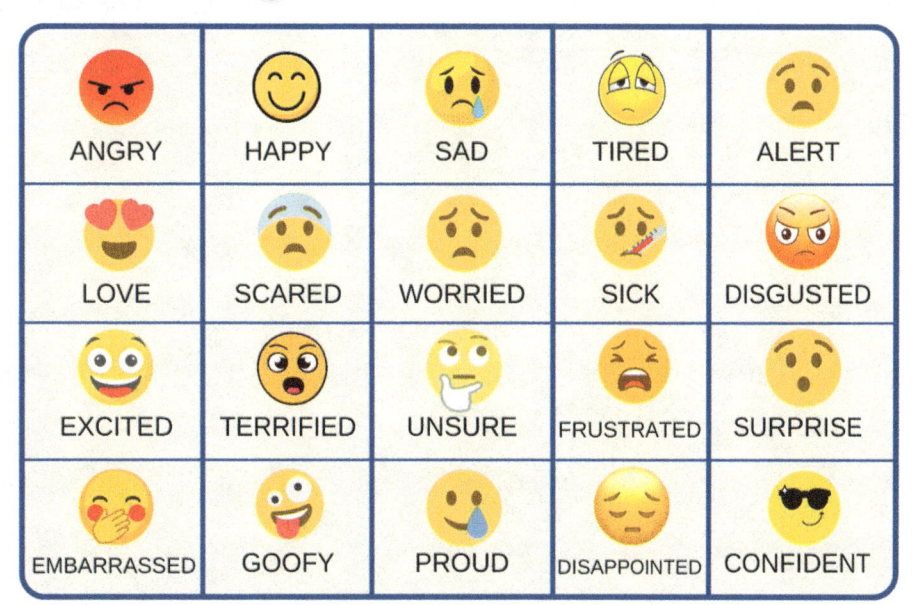

ANGRY	HAPPY	SAD	TIRED	ALERT
LOVE	SCARED	WORRIED	SICK	DISGUSTED
EXCITED	TERRIFIED	UNSURE	FRUSTRATED	SURPRISE
EMBARRASSED	GOOFY	PROUD	DISAPPOINTED	CONFIDENT

Activity Worksheet

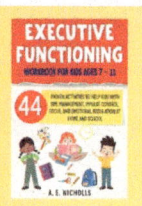

Chapter 4 — Emotional Regulation

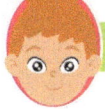

Activity: Breathing Techniques for Emotional Control

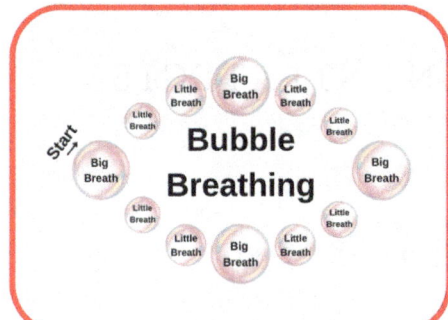

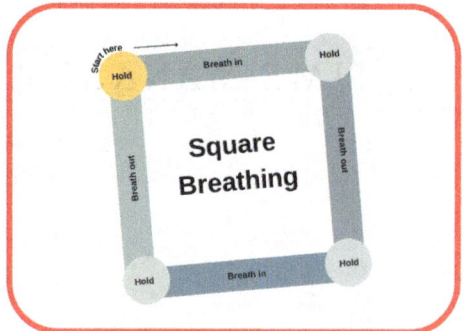

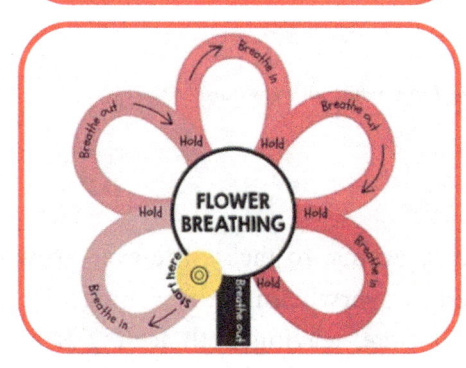

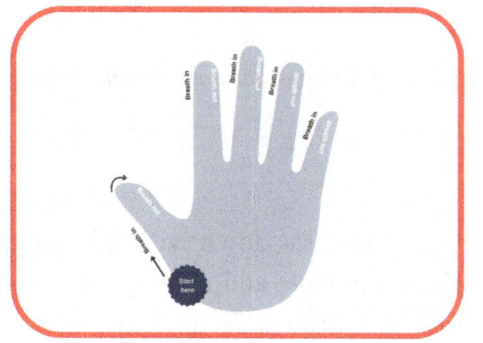

- Bubble Breathing
- Square Breathing
- Flower Breathing
- Hand Breathing

Breathing Techniques Log:

Date	Technique Tried	How I Felt Afterwards

5

TIME MANAGEMENT STRATEGIES

"Time management is not about doing more, but about doing what matters most."

— STEPHEN COVEY

One evening, Sarah sat down with her daughter, Emma, to tackle the ever-growing list of homework assignments and chores that seemed to overwhelm their evenings. Despite their best efforts, they always seemed to run out of time, leaving both feeling frustrated and stressed. Sarah realized that what Emma needed was not just more time but a better way to manage it.

5.1 CREATING A DAILY SCHEDULE

Creating a daily schedule can be a game changer. A well-structured schedule provides the structure and routine children need to manage their time effectively. It helps them understand the concept of time by breaking the day into manageable chunks. This structure reduces anxiety by setting clear expectations, making it easier for children to transition from one activity to the next. Additionally, a daily schedule encourages independence and responsibility. When children know what to expect and when to expect it, they can take ownership of their time and tasks, which boosts their confidence and self-esteem.

Designing a child-friendly schedule involves a few key principles to ensure it is easy for them to follow. Use simple language and visual aids to make the schedule accessible. For instance, a picture of a toothbrush next to "Brush Teeth" or a book next to "Reading Time" can help younger children grasp their tasks. Include time slots for different activities such as school, homework, playtime, and meals. This segmentation helps children understand how their day is divided and what they should be focusing on at any given time. Flexibility is also crucial. Allow room for adjustments to accommodate unexpected events or changes in routine. Involve your child in the scheduling process. Let them have a say in how their day is structured. This involvement fosters a sense of ownership and makes them more likely to stick to the schedule.

For example, a morning routine for a seven-year-old might include waking up, brushing teeth, having breakfast, and getting dressed. Each of these tasks can be represented with pictures and time slots, making it easy for the child to understand and follow. An after-school routine could start with a snack, followed by homework time, playtime, and dinner. This structure ensures that important tasks are completed while still allowing time for relaxation and fun. A weekend routine might include chores, family activities, and screen time. By having a clear plan, children know what to expect, which reduces the likelihood of resistance and meltdowns.

Reviewing and adjusting the schedule regularly is vital to ensure it continues to meet your child's needs. Conduct weekly check-ins to assess what's working and what's not. This review allows you to make necessary changes based on your child's feedback and evolving needs. For instance, if your child struggles to complete their homework within the allotted time, you might need to adjust the schedule to provide more time for this task. Celebrating successes and making improvements where necessary helps keep your child motivated and engaged. Acknowledge their efforts and accomplishments, no matter how small, to reinforce the positive behavior of following the schedule.

INTERACTIVE ELEMENT: WEEKLY SCHEDULE TEMPLATE

Create a simple weekly schedule template that includes columns for each day of the week and rows for different activities. Include sections for morning routines, after-school activities, and evening routines. Allow space for your child to add their own tasks and activities, making the schedule personalized and engaging.

By implementing a daily schedule, you provide your child with the structure and routine they need to manage their time effectively. This practice not only helps them understand the concept of time but also reduces anxiety, encourages independence, and fosters responsibility. Regularly reviewing and adjusting the schedule ensures it remains relevant and effective, helping your child succeed in managing their daily activities.

5.2 FUN WITH TIMERS

Timers are a fantastic tool for managing tasks and activities, especially for children. They create a sense of urgency and focus, making mundane tasks more engaging. When a timer is set, children understand that they have limited time to complete an activity, which helps them stay on task and avoid distractions. This sense of urgency encourages self-discipline and time awareness. Additionally, using timers can turn chores and tasks into fun challenges, transforming what might be seen as boring into something exciting and competitive.

There are various types of timers that you can use to introduce this concept. Digital kitchen timers are straightforward and easy to use. You can set the exact amount of time needed for a task, and the timer will beep when time is up. Sand timers are another excellent option. Watching the sand trickle down can be mesmerizing and helps children visualize the passage of time. Timer apps on smartphones or tablets offer a high-tech solution. Many apps come with fun sounds and visuals that can make the timing process more enjoyable. Visual timers with color-coded sections are particularly useful for younger children. These timers change color as time passes, providing a clear and visual representation of how much time is left.

Incorporating timers into daily activities can make a significant difference in how children manage their time. For instance, you can set a timer for 10 minutes for speed cleaning. Challenge your child to tidy up their room within that time frame. This not only makes cleaning more fun but also teaches them to work efficiently. Homework sprints are another great way to use timers. Set a timer for 15 minutes and encourage your child to focus solely on their homework during that period, followed by a 5-minute break. This method, known as the Pomodoro Technique, can improve focus and productivity. Reading challenges can also benefit from timers. Ask your child to read as many pages as possible within a set time, turning reading into an exciting game. For managing screen time or playtime, use a timer to set limits. This helps children understand how long they have for these activities and encourages them to make the most of their time.

Your involvement in these timer-based activities is crucial. Participate in the activities with your child to make the experience more enjoyable and collaborative. For example, join them in a speed cleaning challenge and see who can tidy up the fastest. Providing positive reinforcement for completing tasks on time is also essential. Praise their efforts and celebrate their successes, no matter how small. This positive feedback reinforces the benefits of using timers and encourages them to continue practicing good time management. Additionally, consider using timers for family activities and games. Setting a timer for a board game or a family workout session can make these activities more structured and enjoyable.

Imagine setting a timer for a 10-minute speed-cleaning session. You and your child race against the clock to see who can tidy up the most within the time limit. The timer beeps, signaling the end of the challenge, and you both take a moment to admire the clean room. Your child feels a sense of accomplishment and learns that cleaning doesn't have to be a tedious task. Or think about a homework sprint, where your child focuses intensely on their homework for 15 minutes, knowing they will get a break afterward. The timer helps them stay on track, and the promise of a break keeps them motivated.

Using timers as a tool for managing tasks and activities offers numerous benefits. They create a sense of urgency and focus, help children understand the passage of time, and turn mundane tasks into fun challenges. By incorporating timers into daily routines and providing positive reinforcement, you can help your child develop self-discipline and time awareness. This practice not only improves their time management skills but also makes daily activities more engaging and enjoyable.

5.3 THE TASK PRIORITIZATION GAME

Understanding how to prioritize tasks is a vital skill for children. It helps them focus on what needs to be done first, reducing the chaos that can come from trying to tackle everything at once. By breaking down tasks into manageable steps, prioritization reduces stress and makes large projects seem less overwhelming. This skill also teaches children decision-making and time management as they learn to evaluate which tasks are most important and why. Completing high-priority tasks first can also encourage a sense of accomplishment, motivating them to continue working through their list.

To introduce the Task Prioritization Game, start by creating a list of tasks with varying levels of importance. Write each task on a separate card or slip of paper. The tasks can range from school-related activities like studying for a test and completing homework to home-related chores such as cleaning their room and feeding the pets. Include extracurricular activities like practicing the piano, attending soccer practice, and finishing an art project. Once you have your list, ask your child to arrange the tasks in order of priority.

Engage them in a discussion about their choices to understand their thought process. For example, why did they place studying for a test before completing homework? This conversation can provide valuable insights into how they perceive their responsibilities and manage their time. Offer guidance if necessary, helping them understand why certain tasks should take precedence over others. For instance, if a test is scheduled for the next day, studying for it might be more urgent than practicing the piano, which could be done later.

You can make the Task Prioritization Game more engaging by incorporating different scenarios. For a school-related task list, you might include tasks like studying for a test, completing homework, and packing a school bag. Ask your child which task they think should come first and why. Discuss the importance of being prepared for the next school day and how packing the school bag can prevent a morning rush. For home-related tasks, you might have cleaning their room, feeding pets, and helping with dinner. Encourage your child to think about the needs of others, such as feeding pets, which might take precedence over cleaning their room.

Extracurricular activities can also be prioritized. If your child has to practice the piano, attend soccer practice, and finish an art project, ask them to consider deadlines and commitments. Soccer practice might have a fixed schedule, while the art project might have a more flexible deadline. Discussing these factors helps your child learn to weigh different aspects of their tasks and make informed decisions.

After playing the Task Prioritization Game, encourage reflection and discussion. Ask your child how they felt about their choices. Did they find it difficult to decide which task should come first? What criteria did they use to make their decisions? Discuss what went well and what could be improved. For instance, if they struggled to prioritize tasks, explore why that was and how they can approach it differently next time. Reinforce the importance of focusing on high-priority tasks first, helping them understand that completing these tasks can make the rest of their workload more manageable.

REFLECTION SECTION: TASK PRIORITIZATION JOURNAL

Encourage your child to keep a task prioritization journal. Each week, have them list their tasks and priorities, then reflect on how well they managed their time. Did they complete high-priority tasks first? What challenges did they face? This practice can help them develop a habit of thoughtful prioritization and continuous improvement.

The Task Prioritization Game is a practical and engaging way to teach children how to manage their tasks effectively. By understanding which tasks need to be done first, they can reduce stress, make better decisions, and experience a sense of accomplishment. Your involvement in discussing and guiding their choices is crucial in helping them develop these essential skills.

5.4 GOAL SETTING FOR KIDS

Setting goals is a powerful way to help children manage their time more effectively. Goals provide a clear direction and purpose, making it easier for kids to understand what they need to achieve. By breaking down larger tasks into achievable steps, goal setting can make daunting projects seem more manageable. This approach encourages motivation and perseverance, as children can see their progress and feel a sense of accomplishment with each step they complete. Tracking progress allows children to celebrate their achievements, reinforcing the positive behavior of working towards their goals.

One effective method for setting goals is the SMART framework. SMART stands for Specific, Measurable, Achievable, Relevant, and Time-bound. This framework helps children create clear and realistic goals. A Specific goal clearly defines what they want to achieve. For example, instead of saying, "I want to be better at math," a specific goal would be, "I want to improve my multiplication skills." Measurable goals allow children to track their progress and see how far they've come. An example of a measurable goal might be, "I will complete five multiplication worksheets each week." Achievable goals ensure that the objectives set are realistic and attainable, given the child's current abilities and resources. Relevant goals are important and meaningful to the child, ensuring they stay motivated and engaged. Time-bound goals have a deadline, which helps children stay focused and provides a sense of urgency.

Consider these examples of SMART goals for different areas of your child's life. For an academic goal, you might set, "I will read one chapter of a book every night for two weeks." This goal is specific, measurable, achievable, relevant, and time-bound. A personal goal could be, "I will practice my piano for 20 minutes every day for a month." This goal encourages daily practice and helps the child improve their skills over time. A social goal might be, "I will invite a friend over to play once a week for the next four weeks." This goal promotes social interaction and helps the child build relationships.

Tracking and reviewing goals is good to ensure that children stay on track and make adjustments as needed. One effective method for tracking progress is using goal charts or journals. These tools allow children to record their progress and see how far they've come. For example, a goal chart might include columns for the goal, the deadline, and spaces to mark progress each day or week. A journal provides a space for children to reflect on their experiences, write about their challenges, and celebrate their successes.

Regular check-ins are also important for reviewing goals. Schedule a time each week to sit down with your child and discuss how their goals are going. Ask questions like, "What progress have you made this week?" and "What challenges did you face?" These check-ins provide an opportunity to offer support and guidance, helping your child stay motivated and on track. Based on their progress and feedback, you might need to adjust the goals. For instance, if a goal is too challenging, you can break it down into smaller, more manageable steps. If a goal is too easy, you can raise the bar to keep your child challenged and engaged.

Imagine your child has set a goal to read one chapter of a book every night for two weeks. Each night, they mark their progress on a goal chart, seeing the visual representation of their commitment. During your weekly check-in, they proudly show you their chart, and you discuss the story they are reading. You notice they are excited about their progress and motivated to keep going. This simple practice reinforces the importance of setting and achieving goals, helping your child develop valuable time management skills.

Encouraging your child to set and track goals not only helps them manage their time more effectively but also teaches them important life skills. By using the SMART framework, tracking progress, and regularly reviewing goals, you provide your child with the tools they need to succeed in various areas of their life. This practice fosters a sense of responsibility, motivation, and perseverance, setting them up for future success.

In this chapter, we have explored various strategies to help children manage their time more effectively, from creating daily schedules and using timers to prioritizing tasks and setting goals. These tools and techniques provide a comprehensive approach to developing strong time management skills. Next, we will delve into enhancing memory skills, offering practical activities to support your child's cognitive development.

Activity Worksheet

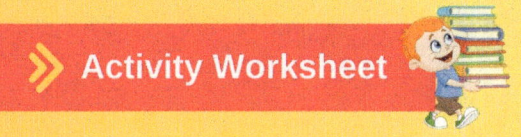

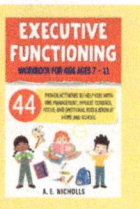

Chapter 5 — **Time Management**

Activity: Creating a Daily Schedule

Chores	Monday	Tuesday	Wednesday	Thursday	Friday	Saturday	Sunday
Morning Routine For example: Brush Teeth	✓	●	●	●	●	●	●
After-school activities	●	●	●	●	●	●	●
Evening Routine	●	●	●	●	●	●	●

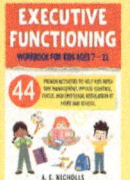

Activity Worksheet

Chapter 5 — Time Management

Activity: Fun with Timers

Instructions:

- Complete each activity below, and time yourself.
- Write down how many times you completed the activity during the time limit. Then, try again later to see if you improve!

Activity	Time Limit	Attempt 1	Attempt 2	Attempt 3
1. How many jumping jacks can you do?	1 minute			
2. How long can you balance on one foot?	30 seconds			
3. How many sit-ups can you do?	1 minute			
4. How many times can you write your name?	1 minute			
5. How long can you hold a plank?	30 seconds			
6. How many times can you toss and catch a ball?	1 minute			

Reflection:

- How did using a timer change how you approached these tasks?

Activity Worksheet

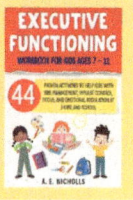

Chapter 5 — Time Management

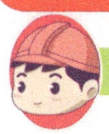

Activity: The Task Prioritization Game

Task List

(Choose tasks from this list and prioritize them in the pyramid below)
1. Study for a math test
2. Complete English homework
3. Clean your room
4. Feed the pets
5. Practice the piano
6. Attend soccer practice
7. Finish your art project
8. Help with dinner
9. Read a book for 20 minutes
10. Water the plants

Instructions:

- Write your tasks in the pyramid below, starting with the most important task at the top.
- The least important task goes in the largest space at the bottom.

Priority Pyramid Worksheet

Top Priority
1. _____

Mid-Level Priorities
2. _____
3. _____
4. _____

Lower-Level Priorities
5. _____
6. _____
7. _____

Lowest Priorities
8. _____
9. _____
10. _____

Reflection:

- Why did you choose this order? How did prioritizing help you complete your tasks?

_____

_____

Activity Worksheet

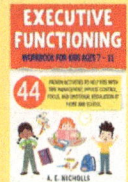

Chapter 5 — Time Management

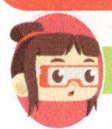

Activity: Goal Setting for Kids

Example Goal:
"I want to read 10 books by the end of the summer break."

SMART Criteria

S - Specific
(What exactly do you want to achieve? Be clear and detailed.)
Example: I want to read 10 chapter books.
Your Goal:
_____
_____

A - Achievable
(Is this goal realistic? Do you have what you need to achieve it?)
Example: I have enough books at home and can go to the library for more.
Your Goal:
_____
_____

T - Time-Bound
(When do you want to achieve this goal?)
Example: I want to finish reading 10 books by the end of summer break.
Your Goal:
_____
_____

M - Measurable
(How will you measure your progress? How will you know you've achieved it?)
Example: I'll keep track of how many books I finish in a notebook.
Your Goal:
_____
_____

R - Relevant
(Why is this goal important to you?)
Example: Reading will help me improve my vocabulary and become a better writer.
Your Goal:
_____
_____

Your SMART Goal

Now, combine everything above and write your final SMART goal here:
My SMART Goal is:
_____

Goal Check-In

Week	What did I do this week?	Am I on track?	Reflection
Week 1		Yes/No	
Week 2		Yes/No	
Week 3		Yes/No	
Week 4		Yes/No	
Week 5		Yes/No	

Final Reflection:

- How did working on this goal help you? What did you learn?

_____
_____
_____

6

ENHANCING MEMORY SKILLS

"The mind is not a vessel to be filled, but a fire to be kindled."

— PLUTARCH

One sunny afternoon, Anna noticed her son, Max, struggling to remember simple instructions while doing his homework. He would forget what he was supposed to do halfway through a task, leading to confusion and frustration. Realizing that this was more than just a one-time occurrence, Anna decided to find ways to help Max strengthen his memory skills. She discovered that memory-matching games could be a fun and effective method to boost Max's short-term and working memory.

6.1 MEMORY MATCHING GAMES

Memory matching games are an excellent way to help children enhance their short-term and working memory, and the kids love playing these games during their OT sessions. These games require children to remember the location of various items or images, which in turn improves their attention to detail and concentration. The interactive nature of these games makes them enjoyable, turning learning into a fun and engaging activity. When children play memory-matching games, they practice recalling information, which helps solidify their memory skills. This process not only enhances their ability to remember but also sharpens their focus, making it easier for them to concentrate on tasks both in and out of school.

There are many types of memory-matching games that you can use to support your child's memory development. One popular type is picture matching with cards. This game involves pairs of cards with identical images, such as animals, shapes, or everyday objects. The cards are laid face down, and players take turns flipping two cards at a time to find a match. This type of game helps children improve their visual memory and attention to detail. Another variation is word and definition matching. In this game, one set of cards has words, and the other set has corresponding definitions. Children must match each word with its correct definition, enhancing their vocabulary and comprehension skills. A third option is object and shadow matching, where children match objects to their corresponding shadows. This game promotes visual discrimination and spatial awareness as children learn to recognize shapes and patterns.

Creating your own memory-matching game can be a fun and rewarding project that you can do with your child. Start by selecting a theme that interests your child, such as animals, shapes, or numbers. Themes make the game more engaging and relatable. Next, make pairs of cards with matching images or words. You can draw the images yourself, use stickers, or print pictures from the internet. Use sturdy paper or laminate the cards to ensure they are durable and can withstand repeated use. Once the cards are ready, store them in a box or bag for easy access. This way, you can pull out the game whenever you have a few minutes to spare, whether at home or on the go.

Playing the memory-matching game is straightforward and can be enjoyed by children of all ages. Begin by laying the cards face down in a grid pattern. The size of the grid can be adjusted based on your child's age and skill level. For younger children, a smaller grid with fewer pairs is ideal, while older children can handle larger grids with more pairs. Take turns flipping two cards at a time, trying to find a match. If a match is found, the pair is removed from the grid, and the player gets another turn. If no match is found, the cards are turned back over, and the next player takes their turn. Encourage your child to verbalize their thought process as they play, such as saying, "I saw a cat here earlier," or "I think this card matches that one." This verbalization helps reinforce their memory and cognitive skills.

INTERACTIVE ELEMENT: CUSTOM MEMORY MATCHING GAME TEMPLATE

To get started, create a custom memory-matching game with your child. Choose a theme, such as "Under the Sea," and make pairs of cards with matching images like fish, shells, and seaweed. Use sturdy paper or laminate the cards for durability. Store the finished cards in a box or bag for easy access. Lay the cards face down in a grid and take turns flipping two cards at a time to find matches. This activity not only enhances memory skills but also provides a fun bonding experience.

Memory matching games are a versatile and engaging way to help your child improve their memory skills. By incorporating different types of matching games and creating your own custom versions, you can keep the activity fresh and exciting. Playing these games regularly will help your child develop better short-term and working memory, attention to detail, and concentration, all while having fun. Please print as many memory matching game cards as you like using the QR code at the beginning of the book.

6.2 STORY RECALL EXERCISES

Recalling stories is a powerful tool for enhancing your child's memory and comprehension skills. When children practice remembering and retelling stories, they improve their auditory memory and listening skills. This process also promotes a deeper understanding and retention of information, as they must process and recall details from the narrative. Moreover, story recall helps develop narrative and sequencing abilities. As children recount events, they learn to organize their thoughts and present them in a coherent and logical order.

One effective way to incorporate story recall into your child's routine is through read-aloud sessions. Choose age-appropriate books or stories that capture your child's interest. Reading aloud with expression and emphasis can make the story more engaging and memorable. As you read, pause periodically to ask questions or discuss key points. For instance, after a significant event in the story, you might ask, "Why do you think the character did that?" or "What do you think will happen next?" These questions encourage your child to think critically about the story and enhance their comprehension.

In addition to read-aloud sessions, there are several activities that can encourage your child to retell stories. One effective activity is to have your child summarize the story in their own words. After finishing a book, ask them to describe the main events and characters. This exercise helps reinforce their understanding and memory of the story. Using props or puppets to act out the story can also be highly engaging. Provide your child with simple props or puppets that represent the characters and key elements of the story. Encourage them to use these tools to reenact the events. This hands-on approach makes the story more vivid and memorable.

Creating a storyboard with key events and characters is another excellent way to help your child recall stories. Provide them with paper and markers to draw a series of pictures that represent the main events of the story. Each picture should depict a different scene or character. Once the storyboard is complete, have your child use it to retell the story. This visual representation helps them organize their thoughts and ensures they remember the sequence of events. It also provides a creative outlet for expressing their understanding of the narrative.

To further reinforce story recall, conduct question and answer sessions after reading. Ask open-ended questions about the story to encourage your child to think deeply about the characters and events. For example, you might ask, "What was your favorite part of the story and why?" or "How do you think the character felt when that happened?" These questions prompt your child to reflect on the story and consider different perspectives. Encourage them to think about the character's motivations and actions. Discussing why characters made certain choices or how they reacted to events can deepen your child's understanding and empathy.

Discussing the sequence of events and any lessons learned from the story is also beneficial. Ask your child to recount the events in the order they occurred. This exercise helps them practice sequencing skills and ensures they understand the progression of the story. Additionally, talk about any moral or lesson the story might convey. For example, if the story involves a character learning the importance of honesty, discuss how this lesson applies to real-life situations. This reflection helps your child connect the story to their own experiences and reinforces the message.

REFLECTION SECTION: STORY RECALL JOURNAL

Encourage your child to keep a story recall journal. After each read-aloud session or story-retelling activity, have them write a brief summary of the story, draw pictures of key events, or answer questions about the characters and events. This journal not only reinforces their memory and comprehension skills but also provides a tangible record of their progress and achievements.

By incorporating these story recall exercises into your child's routine, you can help them develop stronger memory and comprehension skills. These activities are not only effective but also enjoyable, making learning a fun and engaging experience.

6.3 VISUAL MEMORY CHALLENGES

Visual memory plays a crucial role in a child's learning and daily life. When children enhance their ability to remember visual information, they improve their capacity to recognize and recall images, shapes, and patterns. This skill is particularly important in academic settings, where visual cues are often used in teaching materials. Improved visual memory also boosts spatial awareness and attention to detail. These skills are not only vital for subjects like reading and math but also for activities that require keen observation and precision, such as art and sports. When children can remember what they see, they become more adept at navigating their environment and processing visual information efficiently.

One engaging way to improve visual memory is through spot-the-difference activities. These exercises involve providing pairs of similar images with subtle differences. Encourage your child to find and circle the differences between the two images. This activity requires them to closely examine details, enhancing their attention to detail and observational skills. Discuss the differences and how they were identified. For example, you might say, "I see that this tree has three branches, but the other one has four. How did you spot that?" This conversation reinforces their ability to notice small details and articulate their thought process. Spot the difference activities can be found in books and online resources, or you can create your own using everyday objects and drawings.

Visual sequence games are another effective method for enhancing visual memory. Show your child a sequence of images or objects, and have them memorize the order. After a brief period, ask them to recreate the sequence from memory. You can use themes like colors, shapes, or daily routines to make the game more engaging. For instance, line up a series of colored blocks and ask your child to remember the order. Then, mix up the blocks and challenge them to arrange them back in the correct sequence. This activity helps children practice recalling visual information and reinforces their ability to organize and sequence events. By using familiar themes, you can make the game relatable and fun.

Memory grid challenges offer another way to boost visual memory. Create a grid with various images or symbols, and show the grid to your child for a set amount of time. Then, cover the grid and ask them to recall the images and their placement. This exercise requires children to focus on multiple pieces of visual information simultaneously, enhancing their short-term memory and attention to detail. You can start with a smaller grid for younger children and gradually increase the size and complexity as their skills improve. For example, use a 3x3 grid with simple images like stars, hearts, and circles, and gradually move to a 5x5 grid with more complex symbols. Discussing their strategies for remembering the grid can also provide insights into their cognitive processes and help you tailor future challenges to their needs.

Interactive visual memory apps can be a valuable tool for practicing visual memory skills. Many apps are designed specifically to enhance memory and cognitive abilities in children. Look for apps with positive reviews and educational value. These apps often include games that require children to remember and match images, sequences, and patterns. However, it's important to balance screen time with other activities. While digital tools can be effective, incorporating physical and outdoor activities ensures a well-rounded approach to memory development. Encourage your child to use these apps for a set amount of time each day, and complement their digital practice with hands-on activities like spot the difference and memory grid challenges.

VISUAL AID: SPOT THE DIFFERENCE WORKSHEET

Create your own spot-the-difference worksheet with pairs of images that have subtle variations. Use themes like nature, animals, or everyday scenes. Print the worksheet and sit with your child as they find and circle the differences. Discuss each difference and how they noticed it, reinforcing their attention to detail and observational skills.

By incorporating visual memory exercises into your child's routine, you can help them develop essential skills that support their academic and daily life. These activities are not only effective but also enjoyable, making learning a fun and engaging experience for both you and your child.

6.4 REMEMBERING SEQUENCES

Sequential memory is crucial for children as it underpins their ability to follow instructions and complete tasks efficiently. This type of memory involves recalling the order in which things happen, which is vital for understanding and performing everyday activities. In academics, sequential memory supports reading comprehension and math problem-solving. For instance, when reading, children need to remember the sequence of events to understand the storyline fully. In math, solving problems often requires following a series of steps in the correct order. Additionally, sequential memory aids in managing daily routines and organizational skills, helping children navigate their day smoothly and independently.

One fun way to enhance sequential memory is through games that incorporate sequences of actions. "Simon Says" is a classic game that can not only be used to improve instruction-following skills, as discussed in Chapter 3 but it can be adapted to focus on sequences as well. Instead of simple commands, give instructions that involve multiple steps, such as "Simon says, touch your nose, then hop on one foot, and clap your hands." This variation requires children to remember and execute a series of actions in the correct order. Another effective game is number or letter sequencing puzzles. These puzzles involve arranging numbers or letters in a specific sequence, such as putting numbers in ascending order or alphabetizing letters. Completing these puzzles helps children practice their ability to recognize and recall sequences.

Memory chains are another engaging activity for enhancing sequential memory. In this game, each player adds an item to a growing list, and the next player must remember and recite all the previous items before adding their own. For example, the first player might say, "I went to the store and bought an apple." The next player would say, "I went to the store and bought an apple and a banana." This continues, with each player adding a new item while remembering the entire sequence. This game not only strengthens memory but also promotes teamwork and listening skills.

Incorporating sequencing into daily routines can further support your child's memory development. Creating a visual schedule of morning or bedtime routines helps children understand and remember the order of tasks they need to complete. For example, a morning routine schedule might include images representing brushing teeth, getting dressed, eating breakfast, and packing a school bag. Having children arrange routine steps in the correct order reinforces their understanding of sequences. Sequencing cards can be particularly useful for activities like getting dressed or preparing a snack. Provide cards with images of each step, such as putting on socks, then shoes, or spreading peanut butter before adding jelly. Ask your child to place the cards in the correct order and follow the sequence to complete the task. I love how the same strategies work on multiple different Executive functioning skills!

Music and rhythm activities are also effective for improving sequential memory. Clapping or tapping out rhythms and repeating them helps children practice recognizing and recalling patterns. Start with simple rhythms and gradually increase the complexity as your child becomes more comfortable. Learning and performing simple songs with repetitive sequences is another enjoyable way to enhance memory. Songs like "Old MacDonald Had a Farm" or "The Wheels on the Bus" involve repetitive verses that help children remember the sequence of actions or events. Using musical instruments to follow and create patterns can further support memory development. Provide instruments like drums or xylophones and encourage your child to play and repeat sequences of notes or rhythms.

These activities not only make learning fun but also provide practical ways for children to practice and improve their sequential memory. By incorporating games, daily routines, and music into your child's day, you can help them develop the skills needed to follow instructions, solve problems, and stay organized. Strengthening sequential memory supports their overall cognitive development and prepares them for academic and personal success.

In the next chapter, we'll explore techniques to develop flexible thinking, helping your child adapt to new situations and solve problems creatively.

Activity Worksheet

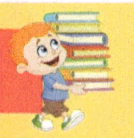

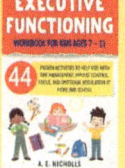

Chapter 6 — Memory Skills

Activity: Memory Matching Games

Instructions:
1. Cut out each card.
2. Create your own matching pairs by drawing or writing on the cards. You can draw objects, numbers, letters, or shapes-anything you like!
3. Once you're done, shuffle them, and they're ready for a memory matching game!

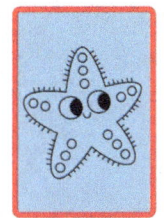

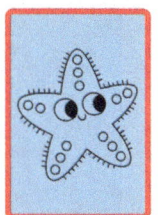

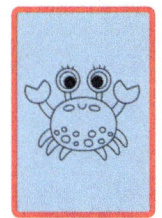

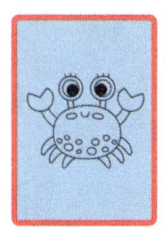

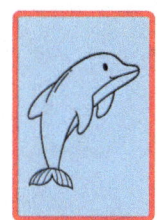

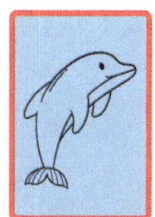

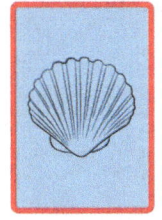

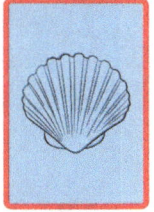

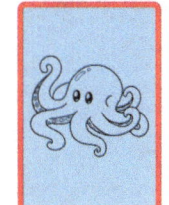

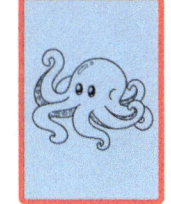

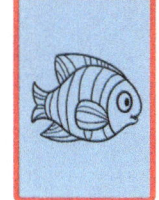

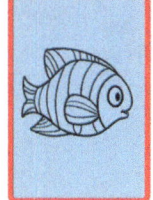

Match Tracking Sheet

Round	Time Taken (Minutes/Seconds)	Matches Found
Round 1		
Round 2		
Round 3		
Round 4		
Round 5		

Reflection Area

- What strategies helped you remember card positions?

Activity Worksheet

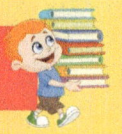

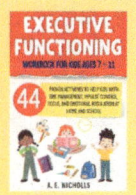

Chapter 6 — Memory Skills

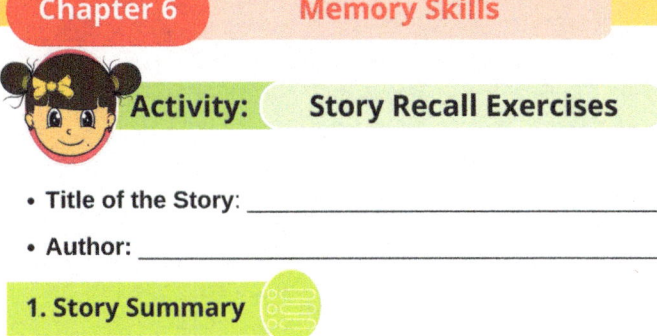

Activity: Story Recall Exercises

- **Title of the Story:** _____
- **Author:** _____

1. Story Summary

- (Write a brief summary of the story. What happened in the beginning, middle, and end?)

  ----

2. Draw a Picture of the Story

- (Use this space to draw a picture of your favorite part of the story, or a scene that stood out to you!)

3. Characters & Events

Main Characters:
(Who are the most important characters?)

Describe a Character:
(Choose one character. What do they look like? How do they act?)

Important Events:
(What were the big moments in the story?)

----

4. Questions About the Story

- (Write down any questions you have about the characters, events, or anything you didn't understand.)
- Why did _____?
- What happened when _____?
- How did _____?

> **Activity Worksheet**

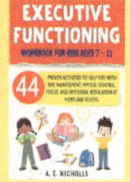

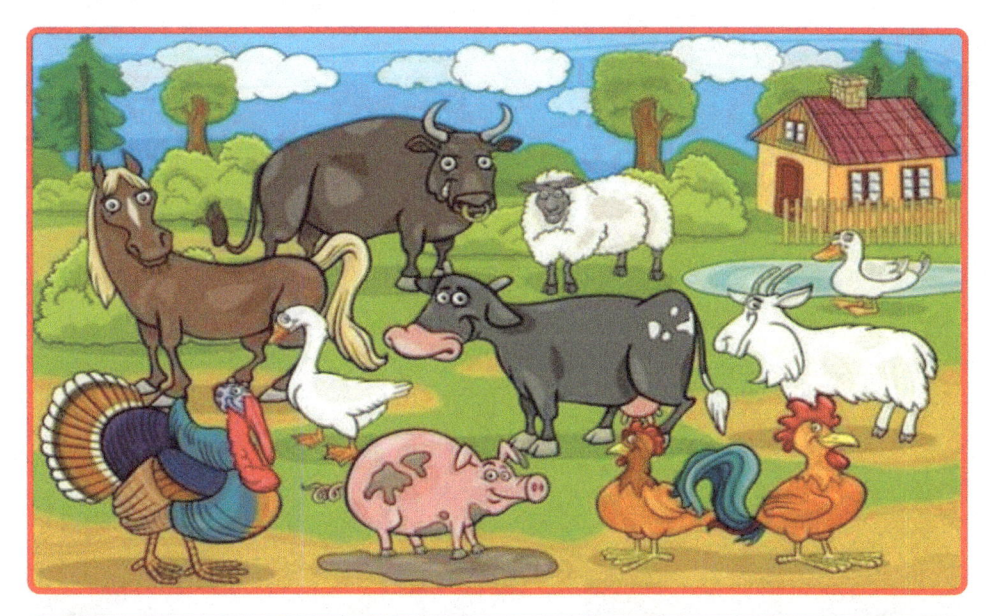

Chapter 6   **Memory Skills**

Activity: **Visual Memory Challenges**

Instructions:

- Look at the two farm pictures closely. There are 10 differences between them. Can you find them all?
- Circle or mark each difference you spot.

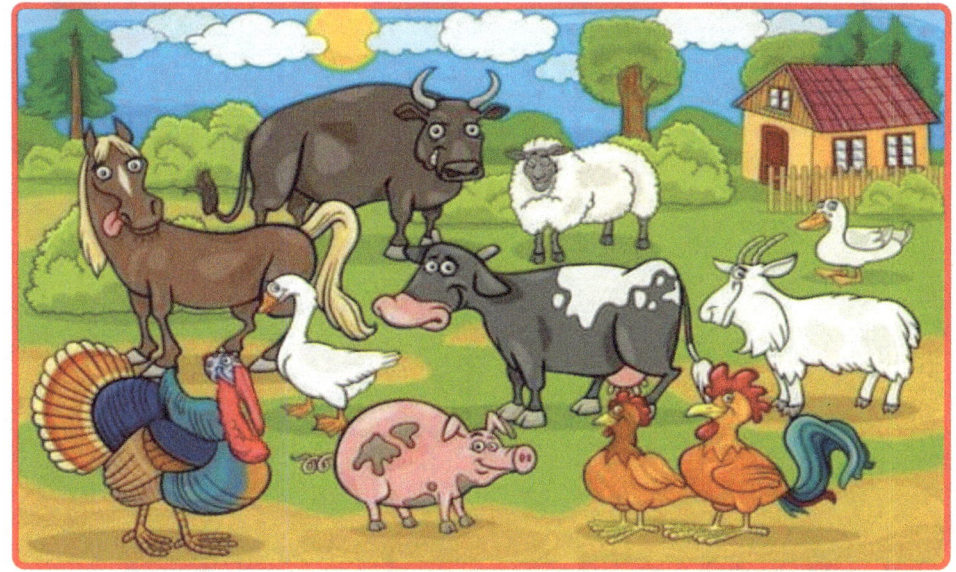

>> **Activity Worksheet**

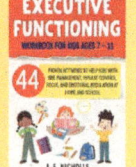

Chapter 6 — **Memory Skills**

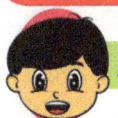

Activity: Remembering Sequences

Instructions:

- Choose a task or process (like brushing your teeth, planting a seed, or baking a cake) and break it down into steps. You can either write or draw each step in the boxes below.

- My Task: _____

Step 1	Step 2	Step 3	Step 4
Write or draw what happens first!	What happens next?	What comes after?	What is the last step?

Reflection:

- How does breaking tasks into steps help you remember them better?

A MOMENT FOR REFLECTION

"Children are likely to live up to what you believe of them."

— LADY BIRD JOHNSON

As we pause in our journey through enhancing executive functioning skills, I hope you've found the strategies and activities shared so far to be valuable in supporting your child's growth. From the Hidden Object Concentration Game to the Calm Down Jar Activity, each tool is designed to make learning fun and effective.

Your dedication to helping your child develop these crucial skills is commendable. The time you invest now will undoubtedly shape their future success and confidence.

If you've found this book helpful, I would be incredibly grateful if you could take a moment to share your thoughts in a review. Your feedback helps others find this resource and contributes to the ongoing conversation about supporting children's executive functioning skills.

Thank you for being part of this journey. Together, we're making a difference in children's lives, one activity at a time.

Now, let's continue exploring more exciting strategies to help your child thrive!

7

DEVELOPING FLEXIBLE THINKING

"Flexibility requires an open mind and a welcoming of new alternatives."

— DEBORAH DAY

Imagine eight-year-old Lucas playing his favorite board game with his family. Just as he's about to win, his dad announces a sudden change in the rules. Lucas hesitates, unsure how to proceed. This moment of confusion is a common scenario for many children who struggle with flexible thinking. Developing the ability to adapt to new situations and think creatively is crucial for navigating the unexpected twists and turns of daily life. Flexible thinking helps children handle changes with ease, solve problems creatively, and view challenges from different perspectives. One effective way to nurture this skill is through the Change-Up Game, which encourages adaptability and quick thinking in a fun and engaging manner.

7.1 THE CHANGE-UP GAME

The Change-Up Game is designed to help children become comfortable with unexpected changes and develop flexible thinking. This game encourages adaptability and quick thinking by introducing sudden changes to familiar activities or routines. By practicing these skills, children learn to handle new situations with confidence and creativity. The game provides a safe and enjoyable environment for children to practice being flexible, which can translate to better coping mechanisms in real-life scenarios.

To play the Change-Up Game, start by choosing a familiar activity or routine that your child enjoys. This can be anything from drawing, cooking, or playing a physical game. The key is to select an activity that your child is comfortable with and knows well. Once the activity is underway, introduce unexpected changes or twists. For example, during a drawing activity, you might switch the drawing tool from a pencil to a crayon. In a cooking activity, you could change an ingredient and ask your child to adapt the recipe accordingly. During a physical game, you might change the rules or objectives midway, such as switching from running to hopping or altering the goal of the game.

Let's delve into specific examples of activity changes. During a drawing activity, start with a simple instruction like, "Draw a tree using a pencil." After a few minutes, announce a change: "Now switch to using crayons and add some animals around the tree." This sudden shift challenges your child to adapt their thinking and approach to the drawing. In a cooking activity, begin by following a basic recipe for making a sandwich. Halfway through, introduce a new ingredient, such as a different type of bread or a unique topping, and ask your child to incorporate it into the recipe. This change encourages them to think creatively and adapt to new circumstances. For physical games, you might start with a game of tag and then announce, "From now on, you can only hop on one foot!" This change requires children to quickly adjust their strategy and movements, promoting flexibility and quick thinking.

Parental involvement is important in the Change-Up Game. By participating in the game, you model flexibility and adaptability for your child. Your engagement shows them that being open to change can be fun and rewarding. Praise your child's ability to adapt to changes, highlighting specific moments where they demonstrated flexibility. For instance, you might say, "I loved how you switched to using crayons so smoothly and added those animals to your drawing!" Discuss the importance of being adaptable and open to new experiences. Explain how flexibility can help them handle unexpected situations in school, at home, and with friends.

REFLECTION SECTION: ADAPTING TO CHANGE

Encourage your child to keep a "Change-Up Journal" where they can reflect on their experiences with the game. After each session, ask them to write or draw about how they felt when the changes were introduced. Did they find it challenging or exciting? What strategies did they use to adapt? Discuss their reflections with them, reinforcing the idea that being adaptable is a valuable skill.

By regularly playing the Change-Up Game and involving yourself in the process, you help your child build the flexible thinking skills they need to navigate life's uncertainties. This game not only makes learning fun but also prepares them to handle changes with confidence and creativity.

7.2 CREATIVE PROBLEM-SOLVING SCENARIOS

Imagine your child faced with a puzzle that just doesn't seem to fit together. They try different pieces, but nothing seems to work. Instead of giving up, they take a step back, consider the picture on the box, and realize they need a different approach. This moment of insight is what creative problem-solving is all about. It's about finding innovative solutions, thinking critically, and being resourceful. Encouraging your child to approach problems from different angles helps them develop these crucial skills, making them more adaptable and resilient in various situations.

Designing problem-solving scenarios for your child can be both engaging and educational. Start by using real-life situations that they can relate to, ensuring the scenarios are meaningful and relevant. Include a mix of simple and complex problems to cater to their developmental level and keep the activities challenging yet achievable. Encourage group discussions and brainstorming to foster collaborative thinking and expose your child to diverse perspectives. For instance, you might ask, "What would you do if you lost your favorite toy in the house?" This scenario encourages them to think creatively about where they last saw it, who might have moved it, and what steps to take to find it.

Consider a scenario where your child needs to work on a group project. Ask them to think about how to divide tasks among team members to ensure everyone contributes and the project is completed efficiently. This exercise teaches them to consider each person's strengths and to communicate effectively with their peers. Another scenario might involve addressing an environmental issue at home. Pose the question, "How can we reduce waste and recycle more effectively?" Encourage them to come up with practical solutions, such as creating a recycling bin chart or organizing a family recycling day. This not only enhances their problem-solving skills but also instills a sense of responsibility towards the environment.

Another valuable scenario involves resolving a playground conflict. Children often face disagreements with their friends, and learning to navigate these situations is crucial. Ask your child how they would handle a disagreement over taking turns on the swings. Encourage them to think about different perspectives and find a fair solution that satisfies everyone involved. This exercise helps them develop empathy, negotiation skills, and the ability to think critically about social dynamics.

Encouraging reflective thinking is an essential part of developing creative problem-solving skills. After your child has worked through a scenario, take the time to ask open-ended questions about their thought process. For example, inquire, "What made you decide to look in that specific place for your toy?" or "Why did you choose to assign that task to your friend?" These questions prompt your child to articulate their reasoning and consider alternative solutions. Discussing the potential outcomes of different choices further reinforces the importance of creativity and persistence in problem-solving.

REFLECTION SECTION: PROBLEM-SOLVING JOURNAL

Encourage your child to keep a problem-solving journal where they can document the scenarios they've worked on, the solutions they came up with, and the outcomes. This journal can include drawings, written descriptions, or even photos of their projects.

Reviewing the journal together allows you to celebrate their successes and discuss any challenges they faced. This reflective practice not only solidifies their learning but also builds their confidence in their ability to tackle new problems creatively.

By providing engaging problem-solving scenarios and encouraging reflective thinking, you help your child develop flexible thinking skills that will serve them well in all areas of life. These activities teach them to approach challenges with an open mind, think critically, and find innovative solutions. Whether they're figuring out how to find a lost toy, collaborating on a group project, addressing environmental issues, or resolving conflicts with friends, they'll be equipped with the skills they need to succeed.

7.3 ALTERNATE ENDINGS STORYTELLING

Alternate endings storytelling is a powerful tool for fostering flexible thinking in children. Encouraging your child to create alternate endings for familiar stories promotes creativity and imagination. It challenges them to think beyond the obvious and explore different possibilities. By considering various outcomes, children learn to understand the impact of different choices and actions. This exercise helps them see that stories, like real-life situations, can have multiple solutions and endings based on the decisions made by the characters.

Choosing the right stories for alternate endings is crucial to making this activity effective and enjoyable. Start with familiar fairy tales or children's books that your child already knows and loves. Stories with clear plots and well-defined characters work best because they provide a solid foundation for creating new endings. Ensure that the chosen story has multiple potential outcomes. For example, classic tales like "Little Red Riding Hood" or

"Goldilocks and the Three Bears" offer rich opportunities for reimagining the characters' actions and the consequent endings.

To guide your child through the process of creating alternate endings, begin by reading the original story together. Discuss the main events and the choices made by the characters. Ask open-ended questions like, "What if Little Red Riding Hood hadn't talked to the wolf?" or "What if Goldilocks had decided to apologize to the bears?" Encourage your child to think about how these changes could lead to different outcomes. Once you've explored some possibilities, invite your child to write or draw their alternate ending. They can create a new conclusion for the story, adding their unique twist to the plot. This exercise not only enhances their creative thinking but also improves their writing and artistic skills.

Sharing and discussing the alternate endings created by your child is an essential part of this activity. Host a storytelling session where your child can share their new endings with family members or friends. This sharing nurtures a sense of accomplishment and boosts their confidence. Discuss the different choices made and their consequences. For instance, ask, "How did your version of Little Red Riding Hood's story change when she decided to take a different path?" Celebrate the creativity and originality of each ending. Praise your child's ability to think outside the box and come up with imaginative solutions.

INTERACTIVE ELEMENT: STORYTELLING SESSION

Organize a storytelling session where children can share their alternate endings with family members or friends. Provide a cozy setting with comfortable seating and perhaps some snacks to make it a special event. Encourage each child to present their new ending and then discuss the different choices made and their consequences. This interactive element not only makes the activity more engaging but also reinforces the concept of flexible thinking.

By engaging in alternate endings storytelling, you help your child develop a more flexible and creative mindset. This activity teaches them to think beyond the obvious, understand the impact of different choices, and explore multiple possibilities. Whether they are reimagining the fate of Little Red Riding Hood or giving Goldilocks a new adventure, they are learning valuable skills that will help them navigate the complexities of real life with confidence and creativity.

7.4 BRAINSTORMING SESSIONS

Brainstorming sessions can be a powerful tool in fostering flexible thinking in children. These sessions encourage open-mindedness and acceptance of different ideas. When children are free to express their thoughts without fear of criticism, they learn to value diverse perspectives. This environment nurtures the ability to generate multiple solutions to a single problem, a key aspect of flexible thinking. Collaborative brainstorming promotes idea sharing, helping children build on each other's suggestions and come up with creative solutions they might not have considered on their own.

To conduct an effective brainstorming session, start by setting a clear and specific topic or problem for your child to brainstorm. This could be anything from planning a family outing to solving a minor household issue. Establish some basic rules to ensure the session is productive. Encourage all ideas, no matter how outlandish they may seem, and emphasize that there is no such thing as a bad idea during brainstorming. Use visual aids like whiteboards or sticky notes to capture each idea. This not only makes the session more interactive but also helps children see their thoughts coming to life. For instance, if the topic is planning a family outing, write "Family Outing Ideas" in the center of the board and let your child add their suggestions around it.

Several specific brainstorming activities can make these sessions engaging and effective. An Idea Web is a great starting point. Begin with a central theme, like "Rainy Day Activities," and branch out with related ideas, such as board games, indoor forts, or baking cookies. This visual map helps children see the connections between different ideas and think more expansively. Another activity is Rapid Fire, where you challenge your child to generate as many ideas as possible within a set time limit. This can be done with a timer and encourages quick thinking. For example, ask, "What can we do with empty cardboard boxes?" and set a timer for two minutes. The goal is to list as many creative uses as possible.

Role Reversal is another engaging brainstorming activity. Ask your child to think from the perspective of a different character or person. For instance, "How would a superhero solve this problem?" or "What would a scientist do?" This shift in perspective encourages children to step out of their usual thinking patterns and explore new approaches. It helps them develop empathy and understand that different people might have different ways of approaching the same problem.

Once the brainstorming session is over, it's time to evaluate and refine the ideas generated. Start with a group discussion to select the most promising ideas. Encourage your child to explain why they think certain ideas are particularly good. This helps them develop critical thinking skills and learn how to evaluate options. Combine similar ideas to create stronger, more comprehensive solutions. For example, if two ideas for the family outing are going to the park and having a picnic, you can combine them into one idea: a picnic at the park. This process teaches children how to synthesize information and build on their initial ideas.

Encourage your child to reflect on why certain ideas were chosen over others. This reflection helps them understand the criteria for good problem-solving and the value of considering multiple perspectives. Ask questions like, "Why do you think this idea will work best?" or "What makes this solution better than the others?" This not only reinforces their learning but also helps them internalize the brainstorming process, making them more adept at it in the future.

By incorporating brainstorming sessions into your child's routine, you foster an environment of creativity and open-mindedness. These sessions teach valuable skills in generating, evaluating, and refining ideas, which are essential for flexible thinking. Whether you're planning a family outing, solving a household issue, or simply exploring new ideas, brainstorming can make the process enjoyable and educational for your child.

>> **Activity Worksheet**

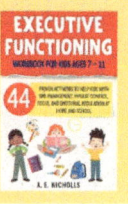

Chapter 7 — Flexible Thinking

Activity: The Change-Up Game

Activity:
(What did you do in the Change-Up game?)

Example: Draw a tree using a pencil, then switch to crayons and add animals around the tree.

1. How Did You Feel?

(Write or draw how you felt when the change was introduced. Did you find it exciting, fun, or challenging?)

Before the Change	After the Change
Write or draw How did you feel before the change-up?	How did you feel after the new challenge was added?

2. What Strategies Did You Use to Adapt?

- (What did you do to adapt to the change? Did you have to think differently, go slower, or be more creative?)

----

3. Reflection:

- Did you find the change challenging or exciting? Why?

- How do you think practicing change-ups can help you in other activities?

Activity Worksheet

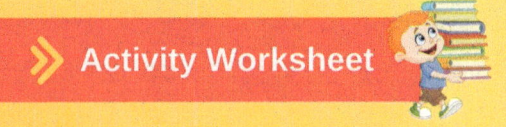

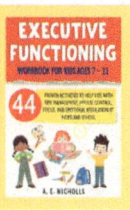

Chapter 7 — Flexible Thinking

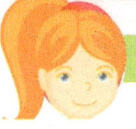

Activity: Creative Problem-Solving Scenarios

Problem Description
(Describe the problem in detail)
Problem:
_____
_____
_____

Proposed Solutions
(List possible solutions to the problem)

Solution 1:
_____
_____

Solution 2:
_____
_____

Solution 3:
_____
_____

Outcomes
(Describe the expected outcomes for each solution)

Outcome of Solution 1:
_____
_____

Outcome of Solution 2:
_____
_____

Outcome of Solution 3:
_____
_____

Visual Representation

- (Add drawings, photos, or diagrams to represent the problem and solutions)

Drawing/Photo:

Reflection:

- (Which solution do you think is best and why?)

_____
_____

Activity Worksheet

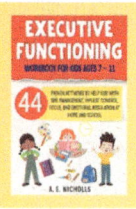

Chapter 7 — Flexible Thinking

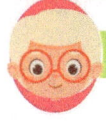

Activity: Alternate Endings Storytelling

Storytelling session

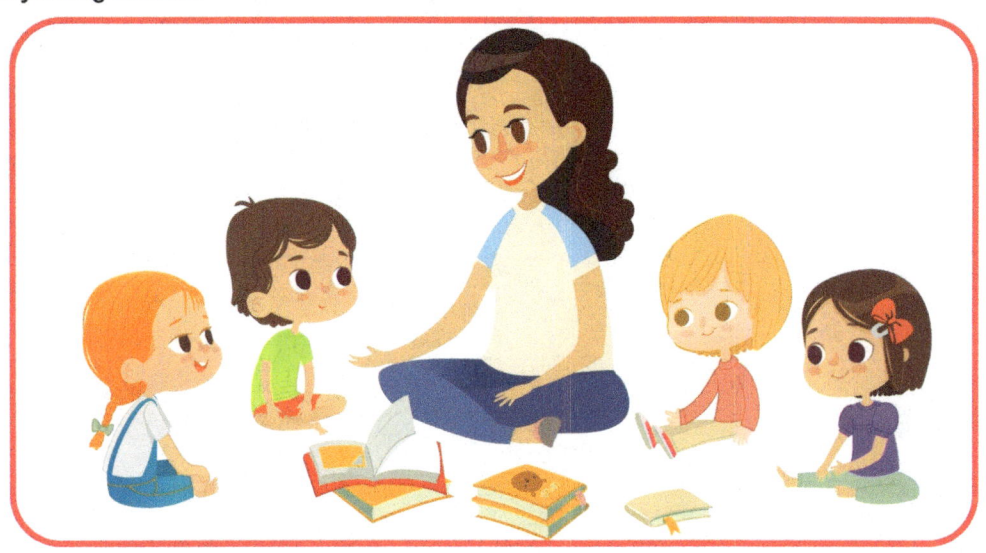

- Organize a storytelling session where children can share their alternate endings with family members or friends. Provide a cozy setting with comfortable seating and perhaps some snacks to make it a special event.

New ending (Write or draw)
For example, "What if Little Red Riding Hood hadn't talked to the wolf?"

Discuss different choices
For example, "How did your version of Little Red Riding Hood's story change when she decided to take a different path?"

Activity Worksheet

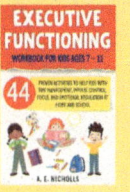

Chapter 7 — **Flexible Thinking**

Activity: Brainstorming Sessions

Mind Map Template

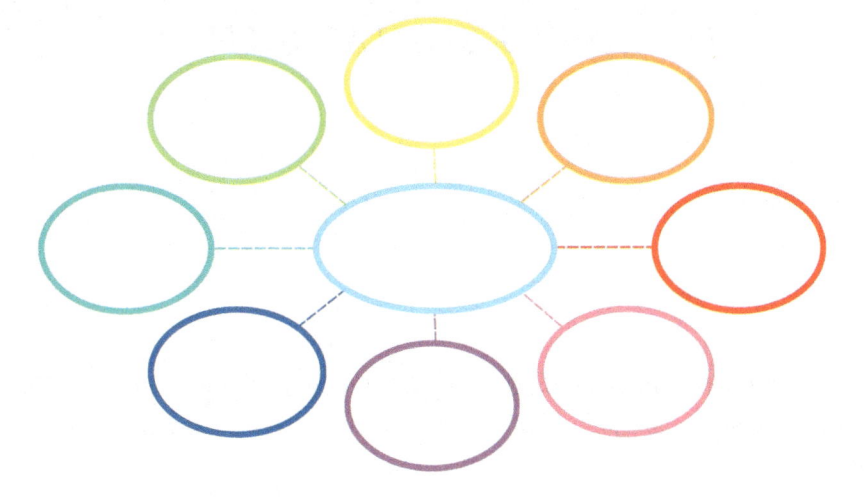

Put a central theme in the middle and branch out.
For example, "Rainy Day Activities," and branch out with related ideas, such as board games, indoor forts, or baking cookies.

Ask reflection questions.
For example "Why do you think this idea will work best?" or "What makes this solution better than the others?"

8

BUILDING SOCIAL SKILLS

"Helping your child build strong social skills is like giving them the keys to a happy and fulfilling life. Through kindness, sharing, and understanding, they can make friends and navigate the world with confidence."

— DR. ROSS W. GREENE.

Eight-year-old Aiden dreaded recess. Every day, he found himself standing alone by the playground, unsure how to approach his classmates. He wanted to join in their games but didn't know how to start a conversation or handle the social cues. For Aiden's parents, watching him struggle with social interactions was heart-wrenching. They knew he was a kind and intelligent boy but lacked the skills to connect with others. Developing strong social skills is crucial for children like Aiden. These skills help them build friendships, work collaboratively, and navigate social situations with confidence. One effective way to nurture these abilities is through role-playing social scenarios.

8.1 ROLE-PLAYING SOCIAL SCENARIOS

Role-playing is a powerful tool for developing social skills in children. It provides a safe and controlled environment where they can practice social interactions without the fear of real-world consequences. By taking on different roles, children learn to empathize with others, understand social cues, and respond appropriately in various situations. For example, when a child plays the role of a teacher or a peer, they gain insight into different perspectives and learn how to adjust their behavior accordingly. This practice helps children build empathy and improves their ability to communicate effectively.

Designing effective role-playing scenarios involves using real-life situations that children frequently encounter. These scenarios should include both positive interactions, such as making a new friend, and challenging ones, like handling a disagreement. This variety ensures that children are prepared for a wide range of social experiences. Encourage your child to switch roles during the scenarios. This role reversal helps them see the situation from different angles, fostering a deeper understanding of social dynamics. For instance, if they role-play as a teacher, they might better understand how to approach a teacher for help in real life.

Consider starting with simple scenarios like meeting a new friend at school. This scenario can help your child practice introducing themselves, asking questions, and showing interest in others. Another useful scenario is handling a disagreement during playtime. This can teach children how to express their feelings calmly, listen to others, and find a compromise. Asking for help from a teacher or adult is another valuable scenario, helping children learn to communicate their needs clearly and respectfully. Sharing toys or resources with peers can also be role-played to practice taking turns and negotiating fairly.

As a parent, guiding the role-play is crucial. Start by providing clear prompts to set the scene and encourage your child to immerse themselves in the role. For example, you might say, "Imagine you are at the playground and see a child playing alone. How would you introduce yourself and invite them to join your game?" During the role-play, offer feedback and encouragement. Highlight what your child did well and gently suggest improvements. This immediate feedback helps reinforce positive behaviors and corrects any misunderstandings.

Encourage discussion after the role-play. Ask your child what they think went well and what could be improved. This reflection helps them internalize the lessons learned during the activity. For instance, after a scenario where they practiced handling a disagreement, you might ask, "How did you feel when you explained your point of view? What do you think you could do differently next time to make the conversation smoother?" These discussions help children process their experiences and apply the skills in real-life situations.

REFLECTION SECTION: ROLE-PLAYING JOURNAL

Encourage your child to keep a role-playing journal. After each session, have them write or draw about what they learned, how they felt, and any new strategies they want to try. Use prompts like, "What was the most challenging part of the scenario?" or "How did you feel when you switched roles?" Reviewing this journal together can provide further insights and reinforce the skills practiced.

Role-playing social scenarios is a practical and engaging way to help your child develop essential social skills. By providing a safe space to practice, offering guidance and feedback, and encouraging reflection, you can support your child in becoming more confident and adept in their social interactions.

8.2 THE TEAMWORK CHALLENGE

When nine-year-old Emily joined her school's soccer team, she was excited but also nervous about working with her teammates. She had always been more comfortable playing solo games and found the idea of relying on others and them relying on her quite daunting. Teamwork, however, is a crucial skill for children to develop. It promotes cooperation and collaboration, enhances problem-solving skills in group settings, and builds trust and mutual respect among peers. Learning to work as part of a team helps children understand the value of shared goals and collective effort, which are important not just in sports but in all aspects of life.

Creating engaging teamwork activities is key to helping children like Emily become more comfortable and skilled at working with others. Start by choosing activities that require collaboration and shared goals. These could be simple tasks like building a tower with blocks or more complex projects like planning a short skit. Make sure the tasks are age-appropriate and achievable to ensure that all participants can contribute meaningfully. Including a variety of challenges keeps the activities interesting and allows children to experience different aspects of teamwork, such as leading, following, and negotiating.

One effective teamwork challenge is building a tower with blocks or other materials. This activity requires children to communicate, plan, and work together to achieve a common goal. They must discuss their ideas, decide on the best approach, and coordinate their efforts to build the tallest and most stable tower possible. Planning and performing a short skit or play is another excellent teamwork activity. It encourages creativity and collaboration as children work together to write a script, assign roles, and rehearse their performance. Completing a group puzzle or scavenger hunt can also be highly effective. These activities require children to combine their skills and knowledge to solve problems and find solutions. Organizing a small event or activity, such as a picnic or game day, allows children to practice planning, delegation, and execution, all essential components of teamwork.

After completing teamwork challenges, it's important to encourage reflection and discussion. This helps children understand their experiences and learn from them. Start by discussing the roles each child played and how they contributed to the group's success. Highlight the strategies that worked well and any areas that could be improved. For example, if a group successfully built a tall tower, discuss how their communication and planning helped achieve that goal. If they encountered difficulties, explore what they could do differently next time to overcome those challenges. Reinforce the value of working together and supporting each other by praising their efforts and emphasizing the importance of teamwork in achieving shared goals.

REFLECTION SECTION: TEAMWORK JOURNAL

Encourage your child to keep a teamwork journal. After each activity, have them write or draw about their experiences, focusing on what they learned, how they felt, and any strategies they found helpful. Use prompts like, "What was the most enjoyable part of working with your team?" or "What was the biggest challenge you faced, and how did you overcome it?" Reviewing this journal together can provide further insights and reinforce the skills practiced.

By engaging in teamwork challenges, children learn to cooperate, communicate, and solve problems together. These activities help them build trust, respect, and a sense of shared accomplishment. With your guidance and support, your child can develop the teamwork skills they need to thrive in group settings and build strong, collaborative relationships.

8.3 EFFECTIVE COMMUNICATION EXERCISES

Effective communication is the cornerstone of building strong social skills in children. When children can express their thoughts clearly and understand others, they reduce misunderstandings and build strong relationships. These skills promote assertiveness and confidence, allowing children to navigate social situations with ease. Clear communication helps children articulate their needs and emotions, fostering better connections with peers and adults. Moreover, good communication skills are essential for resolving conflicts and working collaboratively, both in school and in everyday interactions.

Designing communication exercises for children should focus on both verbal and non-verbal communication. Activities that require active listening and clear expression are particularly beneficial. For instance, partner interviews can be a fun and engaging way to practice these skills. In this activity, children take turns asking and answering questions about each other. This not only improves their listening skills but also teaches them how to formulate and ask questions. Encourage them to maintain eye contact, nod, and use other non-verbal cues to show they are listening. This exercise can be tailored to various topics, from favorite hobbies to future ambitions, making it both educational and enjoyable.

Storytelling with a twist is another excellent communication exercise. One child starts a story, and others add to it, sentence by sentence. This activity encourages creativity and quick thinking while requiring children to listen carefully to continue the story seamlessly. It also helps them practice clear articulation and narrative skills. Emotion charades can further enhance non-verbal communication. In this game, children act out different emotions without speaking while others guess the emotion. This helps them recognize and interpret body language and facial expressions, which are crucial components of effective communication.

Discussion circles can foster open dialogue and exchange of ideas. In a discussion circle, children sit in a group and share their thoughts on a given topic. This setting encourages respectful listening and clear expression of ideas. Choose topics that are relevant and interesting to the children, such as "What would you do if you could be invisible for a day?" or "Describe a time when you helped someone." These discussions not only improve verbal communication but also promote empathy and understanding as children listen to diverse perspectives.

Parental involvement is key to the success of these communication exercises. Participating in the activities alongside your child can model effective communication. For example, during partner interviews, take turns asking and answering questions with your child. Show them how to listen actively and respond thoughtfully. Provide constructive feedback and praise positive interactions. If your child struggles to articulate their thoughts, gently guide them with prompts and encouragement. Highlight the moments when they listen well or express themselves clearly. This positive reinforcement builds their confidence and motivation to practice these skills.

Encourage open discussions about communication experiences and challenges. After each exercise, ask your child how they felt and what they found difficult or enjoyable. Discuss any misunderstandings that occurred and explore ways to improve. For instance, if they struggled with emotion charades, talk about how different body language cues can convey various emotions. These reflections help children become more aware of their communication styles and identify areas for growth.

INTERACTIVE ELEMENT: COMMUNICATION REFLECTION CHART

Create a simple chart to track your child's progress in communication exercises. Include columns for the date, the activity, what they did well, and what they can improve. Use this chart to facilitate discussions and set goals for future exercises. Reviewing the chart together can provide a visual representation of their growth and reinforce the importance of effective communication.

Effective communication exercises are vital for helping children develop strong social skills. By focusing on both verbal and non-verbal communication, encouraging active listening, and promoting clear expression, you can support your child in building meaningful connections and navigating social interactions confidently. Your involvement and feedback are crucial in guiding them through this process.

8.4 SHARING AND TURN-TAKING GAMES

Imagine the scene: eight-year-old Jack is playing with his friends, and a disagreement arises over who gets to use the popular red crayon next. Such situations are common and highlight the importance of sharing and turn-taking. These skills are crucial for social interactions, as they promote fairness and cooperation. By learning to share and take turns, children not only reduce conflicts but also develop patience, which is essential for building a sense of community and teamwork. When children understand the value of waiting their turn, they become more considerate of others' needs and feelings, fostering a more inclusive and supportive environment.

Designing engaging games that teach sharing and turn-taking can be both fun and effective. Choose games that naturally involve these skills, ensuring that the activities are enjoyable and engaging for children. Variety is key to keeping the activities fresh and interesting. For example, board games are an excellent way to emphasize taking turns and following rules. Games like "Candy Land" or "Chutes and Ladders" require players to wait for their turn, teaching patience and fairness in a playful context. Similarly, group art projects can encourage sharing and collaboration. When children work together on a single piece of art, they must share supplies and make collective decisions, reinforcing the importance of cooperation.

Building projects are another great way to practice these skills. Activities like constructing a LEGO tower or assembling a puzzle require children to take turns adding pieces. This not only teaches patience but also enhances their ability to work towards a common goal. Cooperative games, where the focus is on working together to achieve a shared objective, are particularly effective. Games like "The Floor is Lava" or "Human Knot" require children to communicate, strategize, and support each other, promoting a strong sense of teamwork and mutual respect.

As a parent, your guidance and reinforcement play a big role in these activities. Model positive behaviors by demonstrating how to share and take turns during games. For instance, when playing a board game, show your child how to wait patiently for their turn and praise them when they do the same. Provide gentle reminders and encouragement throughout the activity. If a child becomes impatient or forgets to take turns, calmly remind them of the rules and the importance of fairness. This helps them understand and internalize these values.

Discuss the significance of sharing and turn-taking beyond the games. Explain how these skills apply to other areas of life, such as in school, at home, and during social interactions. For example, talk about how waiting their turn in class can help everyone learn better or how sharing toys with siblings can lead to more enjoyable playtime. Reinforcing these concepts in different contexts helps children see the broader impact of their actions and encourages them to practice these skills consistently.

INTERACTIVE ELEMENT: SHARING AND TURN-TAKING CHART

Create a chart to track instances of sharing and turn-taking. Include columns for the date, activity, and specific examples of positive behaviors. Review the chart regularly with your child, praising their efforts and discussing any challenges. This visual tool can motivate children to continue practicing these skills and provide a clear record of their progress.

Encouraging sharing and turn-taking through engaging games is a practical way to help children develop these crucial social skills. By choosing fun activities, modeling positive behaviors, and reinforcing the importance of fairness and patience, you can support your child in building strong, cooperative relationships. Your active involvement and guidance are essential in helping them internalize these values and apply them in various aspects of their lives.

Incorporating these activities into your child's routine will not only enhance their social skills but also prepare them for more complex interactions in the future. As you continue to support their growth, you'll notice improvements in their ability to work with others, resolve conflicts, and build meaningful connections. This foundation of social skills will serve them well throughout their lives, both in personal and professional contexts.

In the next chapter, we will explore strategies for enhancing self-control providing your child with tools to manage their impulses and emotions effectively. This will further support their social development and overall well-being.

Activity Worksheet

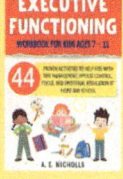

Chapter 8 — Social Skills

Activity: Role-Playing Social Scenarios

1. Scenario: Asking to Join a Game

- **Situation:** You see a group of kids playing a game at recess. You want to join, but they are already playing. How do you ask to join the game?
- **Prompts:**
- What would you say to ask if you can play?
- What if they say "no"? How would you feel?
- What if they say "yes"? How do you show appreciation?

2. Scenario: Sharing Toys

- **Situation:** You have a favorite toy, but your friend wants to play with it. How do you respond?
- **Prompts:**
- How can you share while also respecting your own feelings?
- How would you feel if your friend shared their toy with you?
- What can you do if you don't want to share?

3. Scenario: Dealing with Disappointment

- **Situation:** You didn't get picked for the team you wanted during gym class. What do you do next?
- **Prompts:**
- How do you manage your feelings of disappointment?
- How can you stay positive and still have fun?
- What could you say to encourage yourself?

Reflection:

- Reflection Journal
- Reflection Prompt 1: How Did You Feel During the Role-Play?

- Reflection Prompt 2: What Did You Learn from This Scenario?

Activity Worksheet

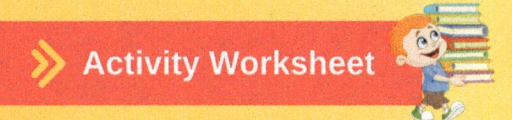

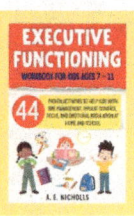

Chapter 8 — Social Skills

Activity: The Teamwork Challenge

Team Members & Roles:

Each team member should have a clear role. List the names of your team members and what they are responsible for:

1. Name:_____
   Role:_____
   Responsibility:_____

2. Name:_____
   Role:_____
   Responsibility:_____

3. Name:_____
   Role:_____
   Responsibility:_____

Steps to Achieve Our Goal:

List the steps your team will take to complete the task or project:

1. _____
2. _____
3. _____
4. _____

Drawing Section:

In this space, draw a picture of your team working together to reach your goal!

Reflection:

- "What was the most enjoyable part of working with your team?"
  _____
  _____

- "What was the biggest challenge you faced, and how did you overcome it?"
  _____
  _____

Activity Worksheet

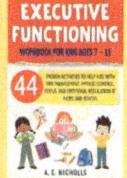

Chapter 8 — **Social Skills**

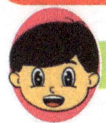

Activity: Effective Communication Exercises

Communication Progress Chart

Date	Activity	What I Did Well	What I Can Improve
[MM/DD/YYYY]	[Describe the activity here]	[Write what went well in the exercise]	[Write areas that need improve-ment or a goal for next time]

How to Use:

- **Date:** Record the date of the communication exercise.
- **Activity:** Briefly describe the activity, such as "Role-playing a conversation" or "Practicing active listening."
- **What I Did Well:** Reflect on your child's strengths during the exercise. Did they maintain eye contact? Did they speak clearly? This column highlights what they did well.
- **What I Can Improve:** Discuss areas for growth, whether it's focusing more on listening, speaking with confidence, or expressing thoughts clearly.

Activity Worksheet

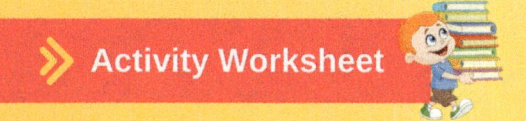

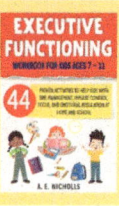

Chapter 8 — **Social Skills**

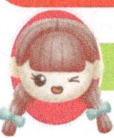

Activity: Sharing and Turn-Taking Games

Sharing & Turn-Taking Progress Chart

Date	Activity	Examples of Positive Behavior
[MM/DD/YYYY]	[Describe the activity here]	[Describe how your child shared or took turns, e.g., "Waited patiently for their turn"]
[MM/DD/YYYY]	[Describe the activity here]	[Example, e.g., "Shared toys without being asked"]
[MM/DD/YYYY]	[Describe the activity here]	[Example, e.g., "Let a sibling play with their favorite toy"]

How to Use:

- **Date:** Record when the behavior occurred.
- **Activity:** Describe the activity where sharing or turn-taking was needed (e.g., "Playing with blocks" or "Board game with friends").
- **What I Did Well:** Reflect on your child's strengths during the exercise. Did they maintain eye contact? Did they speak clearly? This column highlights what they did well.
- **What I Can Improve:** Note specific positive actions your child demonstrated during the activity (e.g., "Asked for a turn politely").

9

ENHANCING SELF-CONTROL

"Teaching children self-control is about giving them the ability to pause, reflect, and make thoughtful decisions. It's a lifelong skill that builds their character and resilience."

— DR. WALTER MISCHEL

One afternoon, while playing in the backyard, nine-year-old Harry dashed after his soccer ball without looking, almost knocking over his younger sister in the process. His mother, Laura, realized that Harry needed to learn how to control his impulses better. Impulse control and self-regulation are crucial skills that help children pause and think before acting. These abilities can be developed through various activities, one of which is the Freeze Game. This game not only enhances impulse control but also provides a fun and interactive way for children to practice self-control.

9.1 THE FREEZE GAME

The Freeze Game is a simple yet highly effective activity designed to help children enhance their self-regulation skills. By requiring children to stop their movements suddenly, the game encourages them to pause and think before acting. This pause helps them develop impulse control, making it easier for them to manage their actions in various situations. The Freeze Game is not just about staying still; it also promotes mindfulness as children become more aware of their movements and the need to control them.

To play the Freeze Game, you need a signal to start and stop the game. This signal could be music, a whistle, or even a simple clap. When the signal is on, children are free to move around and engage in various activities. The key is to let them move freely, encouraging different types of movements like running, jumping, or even dancing. When the signal stops, children must freeze in place immediately. The challenge is to stay perfectly still until the signal starts again. If a child moves during the freeze, they must sit out for the next round. This rule adds an element of consequence, reinforcing the importance of self-control.

The Freeze Game can be adapted in many ways to keep it interesting and challenging. One variation is themed freezes. For example, you can ask children to freeze like a statue, an animal, or a specific shape. This adds a creative twist and makes the game more engaging. Another variation involves adding challenges like balancing an object while freezing. You could have children balance a book on their head or hold a small ball in their hand. These added tasks require extra focus and control, making the game more challenging and beneficial.

Incorporating different types of movements can also keep the game fresh. Instead of just running or walking, you can introduce hopping, skipping, or even dancing. These varied movements not only make the game fun but also help children develop a wider range of motor skills. The more diverse the activities, the more opportunities children have to practice self-control in different contexts.

Parental involvement in the Freeze Game is necessary for reinforcing the lessons it teaches. Playing the game during family time can turn it into a bonding activity that everyone enjoys. As you participate, you can model good self-control and provide positive reinforcement. Observing moments when your child successfully freezes and stays still is important. Praise these moments to encourage their efforts. Discussing the importance of pausing and thinking before acting can further reinforce the lessons learned during the game. Explain how this skill can help them in other areas of life, such as waiting their turn in class or controlling their reactions during conflicts.

INTERACTIVE ELEMENT: FREEZE GAME JOURNAL

Encourage your child to keep a Freeze Game Journal. After each session, have them write or draw about their experience. They can note what movements they enjoyed, what was challenging, and how they felt when they successfully froze in place. This reflective practice helps solidify the skills they are developing and provides a record of their progress. Reviewing the journal together can also offer opportunities for further discussion and reinforcement of self-control techniques.

Through the Freeze Game, children can develop better self-regulation and impulse control in a fun and engaging way. By incorporating variations and involving parents, this simple activity becomes a powerful tool for enhancing self-control.

9.2 IMPULSE CONTROL STORIES

Stories are powerful tools for teaching children about impulse control. They provide relatable examples of impulse control in action, helping children understand the consequences of impulsive behaviors. When children see characters in stories navigate similar challenges, they can better grasp the importance of pausing and thinking before acting. Moreover, these narratives create opportunities for reflection and discussion about self-control, making the lessons more impactful.

To choose appropriate stories for teaching impulse control, look for age-appropriate books with clear messages. Stories that feature characters demonstrating self-control are particularly effective. These characters can serve as role models, showing children how to handle situations that require patience and restraint. Additionally, it's valuable to include stories that show both positive and negative outcomes of impulsive behavior. This contrast helps children see the benefits of self-control and the potential pitfalls of acting without thinking.

For example, consider a story about a character who waits their turn and is rewarded. This type of narrative can illustrate the benefits of patience and the positive outcomes that come from waiting. Another effective story might be a tale of a character who acts impulsively and faces consequences. Such a narrative can help children understand the importance of thinking before acting, as they see firsthand the negative repercussions of impulsive behavior. A third example could be a narrative where a character learns to pause and think before acting, showing the growth and benefits of developing self-control.

Engaging children in discussions and activities related to these stories can further reinforce the lessons. After reading a story, ask questions about the character's actions and their consequences. Encourage your child to think about what the character did right or wrong and how they might handle a similar situation. Questions like, "Why do you think the character decided to wait?" or "What happened because the character didn't think before acting?" can prompt deeper reflection.

Encourage children to share similar experiences from their own lives. This personal connection helps them see the relevance of the story to their everyday actions. For instance, if the story was about waiting for a turn, ask your child if they've ever had to wait for something and how it made them feel. Discussing these personal experiences can help children relate the lessons from the story to their own behavior.

Follow-up activities like drawing or writing about ways to practice self-control can be both fun and educational. Ask your child to draw a scene from the story where the character demonstrated self-control or to write a short story of their own where they practice waiting or thinking before acting. These creative activities reinforce the lessons and provide a tangible way for children to express their understanding of impulse control.

REFLECTION SECTION: STORY DISCUSSION PROMPTS

Use these prompts to engage your child in thoughtful discussions after reading stories about impulse control. "What did the character do when faced with a challenge?" "How did waiting or thinking before acting help the character?" "Can you think of a time when you had to wait for something? How did it feel?" "What would you have done differently if you were the character?"

These discussions and activities not only reinforce the lessons from the stories but also help children develop critical thinking and self-reflection skills. By using stories as a tool for teaching impulse control, you provide children with relatable examples and practical strategies for managing their own behavior.

9.3 SELF-CONTROL REWARD SYSTEM

Using a reward system can be a highly effective way to teach self-control to children. Rewards motivate children to practice self-control by offering immediate and tangible benefits for their efforts. This positive reinforcement encourages them to repeat desired behaviors, making self-control a more ingrained habit over time. When children see that their efforts to control impulses lead to rewards, they are more likely to continue practicing self-control. Additionally, a reward system helps children set and achieve specific goals related to self-control. By breaking down the abstract concept of self-control into concrete actions that can be rewarded, children gain a clearer understanding of what is expected of them and how they can succeed.

Designing a self-control reward system involves a few key elements to ensure it is effective and engaging for your child. Start by using a chart or jar to track progress and rewards. A sticker chart, for example, can visually represent achievements and make the process more tangible for children. Each time your child demonstrates good self-control, they earn a sticker to place on the chart. Alternatively, a reward jar can be filled with tokens or marbles. Every time your child exhibits self-control, they add a token to the jar, and once it is full, they receive a reward. This visual progress tracking helps children see their accomplishments and stay motivated.

Setting clear and achievable goals for self-control behaviors is crucial. These goals should be specific, measurable, and realistic for your child's age and development. For instance, a goal might be to wait patiently for five minutes before interrupting a conversation or to complete a homework assignment without getting up from the chair. Clearly define these goals and discuss them with your child so they understand what is expected and feel involved in the process. It is important to choose meaningful rewards that truly motivate your child. The rewards should be something they value and look forward to, ensuring that they remain engaged and excited about the system.

Different types of rewards can be used to keep the system varied and interesting. Small tangible rewards, such as stickers, small toys, or special treats, can provide immediate gratification. For example, a child might earn a sticker for each act of self-control, and after collecting a certain number of stickers, they can exchange them for a small toy or treat. Privileges or special activities, such as extra playtime, choosing a family activity, or a special outing, can also be highly motivating. These rewards offer children something to look forward to and make their efforts feel worthwhile. Verbal praise and recognition are equally important. Acknowledge your child's achievements with specific and positive feedback, reinforcing their efforts and boosting their self-esteem.

Implementing the reward system involves several steps to ensure it runs smoothly and effectively. Begin by explaining the system clearly to your child and setting expectations. Make sure they understand how they can earn rewards and what behaviors are being targeted. Use simple language and examples to illustrate the process. Monitor and record instances of good self-control consistently. This tracking helps maintain accountability and allows you to provide immediate feedback. Each time your child demonstrates self-control, record it on the chart or add a token to the jar, ensuring they see the connection between their actions and the rewards.

Celebrating achievements and providing rewards consistently is vital for keeping your child motivated. When your child reaches a milestone or achieves a goal, celebrate their success with enthusiasm. Present the reward promptly to reinforce the positive behavior. This celebration not only motivates your child but also makes the process enjoyable and rewarding for both of you. Adjust goals and rewards as needed based on your child's progress. As they become more adept at self-control, you can gradually increase the difficulty of the goals to continue challenging them. Similarly, adjust the rewards to keep them exciting and meaningful.

Through the use of a well-designed reward system, you can effectively teach your child self-control while making the process enjoyable and rewarding. By setting clear goals, tracking progress, and providing meaningful rewards, you create a supportive environment that encourages your child to develop and maintain self-control skills. This system not only helps them in the short term but also lays the foundation for long-term success in managing their impulses and achieving their goals.

9.4 PRACTICING PATIENCE ACTIVITIES

Teaching children to practice patience is a crucial part of developing self-control. Patience helps children learn to wait calmly, manage their impulses, and make thoughtful decisions. When children practice patience, they are less likely to become frustrated or act out impulsively. This emotional regulation is key to navigating daily challenges and interactions with others. Moreover, patience encourages delayed gratification, which is the ability to wait for a reward. This skill is linked to better decision-making and long-term success.

Designing activities that help children practice patience can be both structured and unstructured. Choose activities that naturally require waiting or taking turns. For example, planting seeds and waiting for them to grow is an excellent patience-building activity. This process teaches children that good things take time and effort. Each day, they can water the plant and watch it grow, learning to appreciate the gradual progress. Cooking or baking projects are also effective. These activities involve steps that require waiting, such as waiting for dough to rise or cookies to bake. This anticipation can help children understand the value of patience.

Board games that involve taking turns are another great way to practice patience. Games like "Chutes and Ladders" or "Candy Land" require children to wait for their turn, teaching them to manage their impulses and enjoy the game without rushing. Craft projects that require drying time or multiple steps, such as painting or building a model, can also help children develop patience. These activities encourage children to focus on each step and understand that the final result is worth the wait.

Support from parents and encouragement play a significant role in helping children practice patience. You can model patience in your daily interactions and discuss its importance with your child. Explain how waiting calmly can lead to better outcomes and how managing impulses can make tasks more enjoyable and successful. Provide positive reinforcement when your child demonstrates patience. Praise them for waiting calmly and acknowledge their effort. This positive feedback reinforces the behavior and encourages them to continue practicing patience.

Creating opportunities for children to practice patience in daily routines can make a big difference. For example, during meals, encourage your child to wait patiently for everyone to be served before starting to eat. In social situations, teach them to wait for their turn to speak in conversations. These small, everyday practices help children develop patience in a natural and consistent way.

VISUAL ELEMENT: PATIENCE PROGRESS CHART

Create a simple chart to track your child's progress in practicing patience. Include columns for the date, the activity, and a space for stickers or checkmarks. Each time your child successfully demonstrates patience, let them add a sticker to the chart. Reviewing the chart together can provide a visual representation of their growth and reinforce the importance of patience.

By incorporating patience-building activities into your child's routine and providing consistent support and encouragement, you can help them develop the self-control needed to navigate daily challenges. Patience is a valuable skill that can positively impact their emotional regulation, decision-making, and overall well-being.

> **Activity Worksheet**

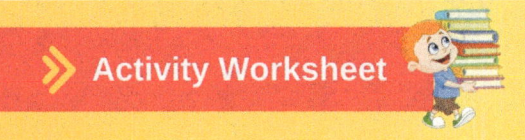

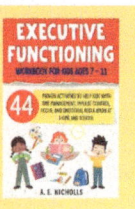

Chapter 9 — **Self-Control**

Activity: The Freeze Game

Freeze Game Journal

This journal is designed to help you reflect on your Freeze Game sessions. After each game, take a few minutes to write or draw about your experience. Think about what movements were fun, what challenges you faced, and how you felt when you successfully froze in place.

Freeze Game Rules:
1. Choose a start/stop signal (music, whistle, or clap).
2. Move freely when signal is on (run, jump, dance).
3. Freeze immediately when signal stops. Hold until it resumes.

Variations:
- Themed freezes (statues, animals, shapes)
- Add challenges (balance objects, specific movements)

Journal Reflection Prompts:

1. What movements did you enjoy today?

----

2. What was the most challenging part of the game?

----

3. How did you feel when you froze in place?

Drawing Section (Optional):

- Use this space to draw a picture of your favorite freeze pose or a fun moment from today's game. Maybe you can show what it looked like to freeze like an animal or hold an object while balancing!

Activity Worksheet

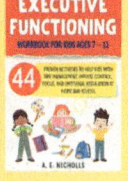

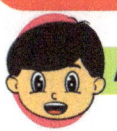

Chapter 9 — Self-Control

Activity: Impulse Control Stories

One sunny afternoon, Jamie was playing in the park with their friends. Suddenly, Jamie noticed a colorful kite stuck in the branches of a tall tree. Jamie really wanted to climb the tree and get the kite down, but then remembered the last time they climbed a tree too fast and hurt their knee. Jamie thought for a moment, looking at the kite and thinking about what to do. Should Jamie climb the tree right away to get the kite? Or should they wait and think of a safer plan?

As Jamie stood by the tree, their friends began cheering, "Go on, Jamie! You can get it!" Jamie felt the excitement but also felt a little unsure. Jamie took a deep breath and...

Story Prompts:

- What did Jamie decide to do next?

- How did Jamie's friends react?

- Did Jamie choose to climb the tree, or come up with another plan?

- What happened at the end of the story?

Reflection

- What did the character do when faced with a challenge?

- How did waiting or thinking before acting help the character?

- Can you think of a time when you had to wait for something? How did it feel?

- What would you have done differently if you were the character?

- How can you apply the lesson from this story in your daily life?

Activity Worksheet

Chapter 9 — Self-Control

Activity: Self-Control Reward System

- **Name :** _____
- **Week of :** _____

How to Earn Stars:

You can earn a star each time you show self-control. Examples of good self-control include:
- Waiting your turn in a game or conversation.
- Thinking before acting in a difficult situation.
- Staying calm when feeling upset.
- Following directions without getting distracted.

Day	Task or Situation	Did I Show Self-control?	Starts Earned
Monday		Yes/No	⭐ _____
Tuesday		Yes/No	⭐ _____
Wednesday		Yes/No	⭐ _____
Thursday		Yes/No	⭐ _____
Friday		Yes/No	⭐ _____
Saturday		Yes/No	⭐ _____
Sunday		Yes/No	⭐ _____

Weekly Reflection:

- What was your biggest self-control victory this week?

- What helped you stay in control when things got hard?

- This chart encourages children to track their progress in self-control daily while reflecting on their biggest success each week!

Activity Worksheet

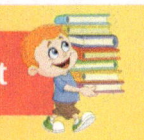

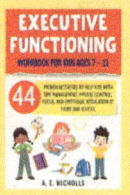

Chapter 9 — Self-Control

Activity: Practicing Patience Activities

- Name : _____
- Week of : _____

How to Use:

Each time you practice patience, you can add a sticker or checkmark to the chart! Here are some examples of practicing patience:
- **Planting seeds** and waiting for them to grow.
- **Baking projects** that take time to finish.
- **Playing games** where you must wait for your turn.
- **Waiting to speak** during conversations instead of interrupting.

Day	Activity	Sticker / Checkmark
Monday		⭐ _____
Tuesday		⭐ _____
Wednesday		⭐ _____
Thursday		⭐ _____
Friday		⭐ _____
Saturday		⭐ _____
Sunday		⭐ _____

Reflection Area:

- How has practicing patience changed your reactions to waiting?

10

PROBLEM-SOLVING SKILLS

"Fostering problem-solving skills in children equips them with the tools to tackle life's challenges with confidence and creativity. Through activities like puzzles and real-life scenarios, kids learn to think critically and persistently."

— DR. CAROL S. DWECK

One rainy afternoon, ten-year-old Alex sat at the kitchen table, staring intently at a jigsaw puzzle. He was determined to finish it, but the pieces just didn't seem to fit. His father, Ben, watched from a distance, marveling at his persistence. He realized that through puzzles, Alex was not just passing time but developing critical problem-solving skills that would benefit him in many areas of life. The ability to solve problems is an essential skill for children, helping them navigate challenges both big and small. Puzzles provide a fun and engaging way to practice and enhance these skills.

10.1 THE PUZZLE CHALLENGE

Puzzles have long been a favorite pastime for children and adults alike. Beyond their entertainment value, they offer significant benefits for developing problem-solving skills. Engaging with puzzles enhances critical thinking and spatial reasoning, requiring children to analyze patterns, shapes, and colors to find the right fit. This process sharpens their ability to think critically and make connections between pieces. Moreover, puzzles encourage persistence and patience. Completing a puzzle can be a lengthy process, but the satisfaction of fitting the last piece is a powerful reward. This teaches children the value of sticking with a task, even when it gets challenging.

The types of puzzles available are varied, catering to different interests and skill levels. Jigsaw puzzles are perhaps the most common, with pieces ranging from simple shapes for younger children to complex images of hundreds or even thousands of pieces for older kids. These puzzles help develop visual-spatial skills as children learn to recognize how pieces fit together to form a complete picture. Logic puzzles, such as Sudoku or crosswords, challenge children to use deductive reasoning to solve problems. These puzzles enhance analytical thinking and improve vocabulary and math skills. Additionally, 3D puzzles or building sets like LEGO offer a hands-on approach to problem-solving. As children construct three-dimensional models, they develop fine motor skills and learn to visualize structures in space.

To organize a puzzle challenge, set up a time-limited puzzle-solving session. Choose a puzzle appropriate for your child's age and skill level. For younger children, a simple jigsaw puzzle with larger pieces can be a good start. Older children might enjoy more complex puzzles or logic challenges. Set a timer for the session, creating a sense of urgency and focus. Encourage your child to work individually or in groups, fostering both independence and teamwork. Offer hints or assistance if needed to keep the challenge engaging but not too frustrating. The goal is to create a balance between challenge and encouragement, helping your child experience success and growth.

After completing the puzzle challenge, take time to reflect on the puzzle-solving process. Discuss the strategies your child used to solve the puzzle. Did they start by finding the edge pieces first? Did they group pieces by color or pattern? Highlight any challenges they faced and how they overcame them. This reflection helps reinforce the importance of persistence and creative thinking. Encourage your child to think about what worked well and what they might do differently next time. This process of reflection not only enhances their problem-solving skills but also helps them develop a growth mindset, understanding that challenges are opportunities for learning and improvement.

REFLECTION SECTION: STRATEGIES AND SOLUTIONS

Create a simple worksheet to help your child reflect on their puzzle-solving experience. Include sections for them to write about the strategies they used, any challenges they faced, and how they overcame those challenges. Discuss their reflections together, reinforcing the positive aspects of their approach and suggesting new strategies for future puzzles.

By incorporating puzzle challenges into your child's routine, you provide them with a fun and engaging way to develop essential problem-solving skills. Puzzles enhance critical thinking, spatial reasoning, persistence, and patience. They also offer opportunities for reflection, helping your child understand and improve their problem-solving strategies. Whether working on a jigsaw puzzle, a logic puzzle, or a 3D building set, your child will gain valuable skills that will serve them well in many areas of life.

10.2 REAL-LIFE PROBLEM SOLVING

Children often encounter various real-life problems that require effective problem-solving skills. These skills are invaluable as they apply to everyday scenarios, enhancing practical thinking and decision-making abilities. When children practice problem-solving in real-life situations, they build confidence in handling real-life challenges. Imagine your child planning a small family game night. This task involves deciding which games to play, organizing the time, and ensuring everyone has fun. By engaging in this activity, your child learns to plan and execute an event, considering the preferences and schedules of all family members.

Another common scenario is organizing a personal space, such as a bedroom or study area. This task helps children develop organizational skills and a sense of responsibility for their environment. They learn to prioritize items, find efficient storage solutions, and maintain a tidy space. Managing a small budget for a shopping trip is another practical problem-solving exercise. Give your child a set amount of money and a list of items to buy. This activity teaches them to make decisions based on available resources, compare prices, and understand the value of money. It also encourages critical thinking as they weigh the importance of different items and make choices accordingly.

Resolving a minor conflict with a sibling or friend is a valuable real-life problem-solving opportunity. These situations teach children to communicate effectively, understand different perspectives, and find mutually beneficial solutions. For example, if two siblings disagree about which movie to watch, guiding them to discuss their preferences, take turns, or find a compromise fosters their conflict resolution skills. Engaging in these real-life problems helps children apply their problem-solving skills in meaningful contexts, making the learning process more relevant and impactful.

Guiding children through real-life problem-solving involves several steps. First, identify the problem clearly and discuss its importance. For instance, if your child needs to organize their study area, explain why a tidy space can improve their focus and productivity. Next, brainstorm possible solutions and evaluate their feasibility. Encourage your child to think creatively and consider multiple options. For example, they might suggest different ways to arrange their books and school supplies. Discuss the pros and cons of each solution and help them choose the best one.

Once a solution is chosen, create a plan of action. Break down the steps needed to implement the solution and ensure your child understands what needs to be done. For instance, if they decide to organize their study area, the plan might include sorting items into categories, finding suitable storage containers, and arranging the space logically. Implement the solution and review the results together. Encourage your child to reflect on what worked well and what could be improved. This reflection reinforces the value of practical problem-solving and helps them learn from their experiences.

Reflection is a crucial part of the problem-solving process. After implementing a solution, take time to discuss the outcome with your child. Ask questions like, "What did you find challenging about this task?" or "What strategy worked best for you?" Highlight the skills they used and their relevance to other situations. For example, if your child successfully organized their study area, point out how the same skills can be applied to organizing their schoolwork or planning a project. Reinforce the value of adaptability and encourage them to keep practicing these skills in different contexts.

REFLECTION SECTION: PROBLEM-SOLVING JOURNAL

Encourage your child to keep a problem-solving journal. In this journal, they can document real-life problems they encounter, the solutions they brainstorm, and the outcomes of their actions. Include prompts like, "What problem did you solve today?" and "What did you learn from this experience?" Reviewing the journal together provides an opportunity to celebrate successes, discuss challenges, and reinforce the importance of practical problem-solving. This ongoing reflection helps your child develop a growth mindset and become more resilient when facing new challenges.

10.3 DECISION-MAKING SCENARIOS

Decision-making is the foundation of effective problem-solving. It helps children evaluate options and make informed choices. Developing this skill encourages kids to think through the possible consequences of their actions. It also builds their confidence in making decisions independently. By providing opportunities to practice decision-making, you help your child become more adept at navigating various situations.

Creating engaging decision-making scenarios starts with choosing age-appropriate and relatable situations. Consider both simple and complex decisions to provide a range of experiences. For instance, deciding between two extracurricular activities involves weighing different interests and schedules. This scenario helps children learn to prioritize their commitments and think about what they enjoy most. On the other hand, deciding how to spend free time effectively might involve balancing play, homework, and chores. This teaches them to manage their time wisely.

Encourage discussion and justification of choices to deepen their understanding. For example, if your child is deciding between joining the soccer team or the art club, ask them why they prefer one over the other. What do they enjoy about each activity? What are their goals? This process helps them articulate their thoughts and consider various factors, such as time commitment, personal interest, and social opportunities. It also teaches them to think critically about their decisions and understand the importance of making informed choices.

Let's explore some specific scenarios that can help your child practice decision-making. Choosing between two extracurricular activities is a common decision for many children. This scenario allows them to evaluate their interests, consider their schedule, and think about what they enjoy doing in their free time. Another scenario might involve deciding how to spend free time effectively. Should they play video games, read a book, or help with household chores? This decision requires them to balance leisure, learning, and responsibilities.

Making healthy food choices at a meal is another valuable scenario. For example, if your child is choosing between a sugary snack and a piece of fruit, discuss the benefits of each option. What will give them more energy? What will help them stay focused during the day? This scenario helps them understand the impact of their choices on their health and well-being. Planning a weekend activity with family or friends is another engaging decision-making scenario. Should they go to the park, watch a movie, or play board games? This decision involves considering everyone's preferences and finding a compromise that makes everyone happy.

Evaluating the decisions made and their outcomes is important for reinforcing learning. Discuss the reasoning behind their choices. Why did they choose to join the soccer team instead of the art club? Reflect on the consequences of their decisions. Did they enjoy the activity? Did it fit into their schedule? Encourage them to think about alternative options and their potential outcomes. For example, if they had chosen differently, how might their experience have changed? This reflection helps them understand the impact of their decisions and learn from their experiences.

REFLECTION SECTION: DECISION-MAKING JOURNAL

Encourage your child to keep a decision-making journal. In this journal, they can document the decisions they make, the reasoning behind their choices, and the outcomes of their decisions. Include prompts like, "What decision did you make today?" and "What did you learn from this experience?" Reviewing the journal together provides an opportunity to discuss their thought process, celebrate successes, and identify areas for improvement. This ongoing reflection helps your child develop a thoughtful and confident approach to decision-making.

Practicing decision-making scenarios is a powerful way to enhance your child's problem-solving skills. By evaluating options, considering consequences, and making informed choices, children develop critical thinking and confidence. These skills are invaluable for navigating the complexities of daily life, helping them become more independent and capable individuals.

10.4 THE LOGIC GAME

Logic games are incredible tools for developing problem-solving skills in children. They offer a fun and interesting way to practice logical reasoning and analytical thinking. Engaging in these games encourages children to recognize patterns and plan strategically, skills that are invaluable both in academic settings and everyday life. For example, when a child plays a logic game, they must think several steps ahead, considering the consequences of each move. This kind of forward-thinking enhances their ability to solve problems methodically and efficiently.

There are various types of logic games that can be beneficial. Classic logic puzzles, such as grid puzzles or riddles, challenge children to use deductive reasoning to arrive at a solution. These puzzles often require them to eliminate possibilities systematically, fostering a disciplined approach to problem-solving. Strategy games like chess or checkers also offer significant benefits. In chess, for instance, children learn to anticipate their opponent's moves and plan their strategy accordingly. This not only sharpens their strategic thinking but also improves their ability to adapt to changing situations. Digital logic games and apps provide a modern twist, offering interactive and engaging ways to develop logical reasoning. Many of these apps are designed to be educational, making learning fun and accessible.

Organizing a logic game session can be an exciting and educational activity for children. Start by selecting a variety of logic games to cater to different interests and skill levels. This ensures that every child finds something they enjoy and can engage with. Encourage individual play to foster independence and self-reliance. Alternatively, introduce friendly competition to add an element of excitement and motivation. You can offer guidance and hints to keep the games engaging and challenging without becoming overwhelming. For example, if your child struggles with a particular puzzle, provide subtle hints that guide them toward the solution without giving it away. This approach helps them build confidence and resilience.

Reflecting on the strategies used in logic games is a crucial part of the learning process. After the game, take time to discuss the thought process behind solving the puzzles. Ask your child to explain how they approached the game and what strategies they found effective. Highlight any patterns or tactics that worked well, reinforcing the importance of logical thinking and strategic planning. This reflection helps children understand their strengths and areas for improvement, fostering a growth mindset. Encourage them to think about how the skills they used in the game can apply to real-life situations, such as planning a project or solving a problem at school.

REFLECTION SECTION: STRATEGY DISCUSSION

Create a simple chart to help your child reflect on their logic game strategies. Include columns for the game played, the strategies used, and the outcomes. This visual aid can help them see patterns in their thinking and identify successful tactics. Discuss the chart together, highlighting what worked well and what could be improved. This ongoing reflection reinforces the skills they are developing and encourages continuous improvement.

Incorporating logic games into your child's routine offers a fun and effective way to enhance their problem-solving skills. These games develop logical reasoning, analytical thinking, pattern recognition, and strategic planning. By organizing engaging game sessions and reflecting on the strategies used, you can help your child build a strong foundation in problem-solving. As they become more adept at these games, they'll find that the skills they develop will serve them well in many areas of life, from academics to everyday challenges.

Activity Worksheet

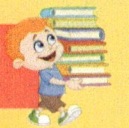

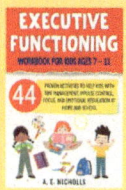

Chapter 10 — **Problem-Solving**

Activity: The Puzzle Challenge

- **Name :** _____
- **Date :** _____

1. What Puzzle Did You Complete?
(Write about the puzzle you worked on, like how big it was or what picture it made!)

----

2. What Strategies Did You Use?
(What steps did you take to solve the puzzle? Did you start with the corners, edges, or sort by color?)

----

3. What Challenges Did You Face?
(Was there a part of the puzzle that was really hard? Did you feel stuck at any point?)

----

4. How Did You Overcome Those Challenges?
(What helped you keep going when the puzzle got hard? Did you try a new idea, ask for help, or take a break?)

----

5. Reflection Discussion

(Discuss your answers with an adult. Think about what worked well and what could be even better for the next time!)

- **What went well with your puzzle-solving?**

- **What new strategies could you try next time?**

Activity Worksheet

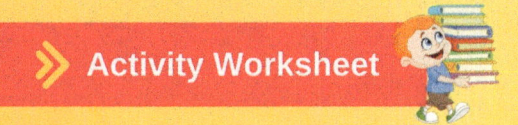

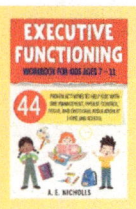

Chapter 10 — Problem-Solving

Activity: Real-Life Problem Solving

- **Name :** _____
- **Date :** _____

1. What Problem Did You Encounter Today?
(Describe the real-life problem you faced. It could be something at school, at home, or with friends.)

----

2. What Solutions Did You Think of?
(List the different ideas you had to solve the problem. Did you think of them on your own or with help from others?)

1. ---
2. ---
3. ---

3. What Solution Did You Try?
(Write down which solution you chose and why you decided to try that one.)

----

4. What Happened?
(Describe what happened after you tried your solution. Did it work, or was it harder than you thought?)

----

5. Reflection Section:

- What problem did you solve today?

- What did you learn from this experience?

- Would you do anything differently next time? If yes, what?

- How do you feel now that you've solved the problem?

Activity Worksheet

Chapter 10 — Problem-Solving

Activity: Decision-Making Scenarios

- Name : _____
- Date : _____

1. What Decision Did You Make Today?
(Describe the decision you had to make. Was it a big decision or a small one?)

----

2. What Were Your Options?
(List the different choices you had. Did you have to pick between a few things?)
1._____
2._____
3._____

Pros and Cons Chart

- Use this chart to weigh the good and bad sides of each option before making your decision.)

Option	Pros (Good Things)	Cons (Not So Good Things)
Option 1:		
Option 2:		
Option 3:		

4. Which Option Did You Choose?
(Which option did you decide to go with, and why did you pick that one?)

----

5. What Happened After Your Decision?
(Describe the outcome of your choice. Did it work out the way you thought it would?)

----

5. Reflection Section:

- What decision did you make today?

- If you could go back, would you make the same decision or choose a different option? Why?

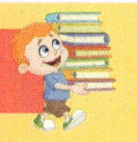

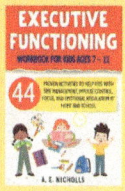

- What did you learn from this experience?

- How can you use this experience to help with future decisions?

Activity Worksheet

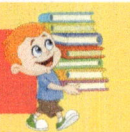

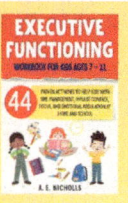

Chapter 10 — Problem-Solving

Activity: The Logic Game

Four friends **Jack**, **Mia**, **Oscar**, and **Lily** each have a different pet: a **dog**, a **cat**, a **rabbit**, and a **parrot**. Use the clues below to figure out which pet each person owns.

Clues:
1. Jack doesn't have a pet that can fly.
2. Mia's pet has fur but doesn't bark.
3. Lily is allergic to fur.
4. Oscar's pet can hop.

Name	Dog	Cat	Rabbit	Parrot
Jack				
Mia				
Lily				
Oscar				

Logic Game Reflection Chart

Game Played	Strategies Used	Outcome
		Success/Struggled Incomplette
		Success/Struggled Incomplette
		Success/Struggled Incomplette

Discussion Section

1. What worked well in your logic game strategy?
(What strategies helped you solve the game faster or with fewer mistakes?)

----

2. What could be improved next time?
(Did you make any mistakes or get stuck? What could you do differently next time?)

11

ENCOURAGING SELF-REFLECTION

"Encouraging children to engage in self-reflection helps them understand their thoughts and emotions, fostering personal growth and emotional intelligence. Simple practices like journaling or drawing can provide a powerful means for them to process their experiences."

— DR. E. SCOTT HUEBNER

One evening, as ten-year-old Lily sat quietly in her room, her mother, Karen, noticed a small notebook on Lily's desk filled with colorful drawings and scribbles. Curious, Karen asked Lily about it, and Lily excitedly explained that it was her journal, where she wrote about her day, her feelings, and the things she learned. Karen realized that this simple act of journaling was helping Lily process her emotions and experiences in a healthy way. This discovery inspired Karen to support Lily in making journaling a regular part of her routine, recognizing its profound benefits.

11.1 DAILY JOURNALING PROMPTS

Introducing your child to daily journaling can be a transformative experience. It's been mentioned a lot in the book because journaling provides a safe space where children can freely express their thoughts and feelings without fear of judgment. This practice enhances self-awareness and emotional understanding, allowing children to reflect on their daily experiences and gain insights into their behaviors and emotions. Regular journaling helps develop writing and critical thinking skills as children learn to articulate their thoughts clearly and analyze their experiences. Also, it encourages a habit of self-reflection, fostering a deeper connection with their inner selves.

When creating journaling prompts for your child, it's essential to use simple and clear language that they can easily understand. Open-ended questions are particularly effective, as they encourage thoughtful responses and allow children to explore a range of topics. Prompts should cover various aspects of self-reflection, including emotions, experiences, and goals. Providing examples can help children get started and feel more comfortable with the process. For instance, you might ask, "What made you happy today and why?" This question encourages children to focus on positive experiences and reflect on the reasons behind their happiness. Another prompt could be, "Describe a challenge you faced and how you handled it." This allows children to think about their problem-solving skills and resilience.

Examples of daily journaling prompts can be tailored to suit different aspects of self-reflection. For example, to help children reflect on their emotions, you might ask, "What is one thing you learned today?" This prompt encourages children to think about their growth and development. Another useful prompt is, "Write about a time when you helped someone. How did it make you feel?" This question promotes empathy and helps children understand the impact of their actions on others. By regularly engaging with these prompts, children can develop a habit of introspection, leading to greater self-awareness and emotional intelligence.

Incorporating journaling into your child's daily routine can be both simple and rewarding. Set aside a specific time each day for journaling, such as before bed, to create a consistent habit. A comfortable and quiet space for writing is essential, as it allows children to concentrate and reflect without distractions. Encourage your child to share their journal entries with a trusted adult if they feel comfortable, fostering open communication and providing an opportunity for further reflection and discussion. Sharing can also help children feel supported and understood, reinforcing the positive impact of their journaling practice.

INTERACTIVE ELEMENT: DAILY JOURNALING PROMPTS PRINTABLE

To support your child in their journaling journey, consider creating a printable sheet with a variety of prompts. This can serve as a handy reference and inspire them to explore different aspects of their thoughts and feelings. Include prompts such as:

- "What made you smile today?"
- "Describe a time when you felt proud of yourself."
- "What is something you want to improve on? How will you do it?"
- "Write about a fun activity you did today."

By providing a range of prompts, you can help your child explore different dimensions of their experiences and emotions. This practice not only enhances their self-awareness but also encourages them to think critically about their actions and decisions. Over time, journaling can become a valuable tool for personal growth, helping your child navigate the complexities of their emotions and experiences with greater clarity and confidence.

11.2 THE SELF-REFLECTION MIRROR

One evening, as your child brushes their teeth, they catch a glimpse of themselves in the bathroom mirror. This moment can be more than just routine; it can be an opportunity for self-reflection and growth. A self-reflection mirror serves as a tangible and visual tool that encourages children to look at themselves and think about their actions and emotions. It can be a powerful metaphor for introspection, helping them understand their feelings and behaviors better. By regularly engaging with their reflection, children can develop a deeper sense of self-awareness, which is crucial for personal growth.

Setting up a self-reflection mirror is simple and can be done with a few thoughtful touches. Choose a mirror that your child can easily access, whether it's in their bedroom, bathroom, or a common area. The key is to ensure it's in a place where they feel comfortable and can spend a few quiet moments each day. Decorating the mirror with positive affirmations and encouraging words can make it more inviting and inspiring. Phrases like "You are strong," "You are kind," and "You can do it" can boost their confidence and motivate them to engage in self-reflection. Placing the mirror in a private, comfortable area ensures they have a safe space to explore their thoughts without distractions.

Daily self-reflection exercises can make this practice more meaningful. Encourage your child to look in the mirror and say three positive things about themselves each day. This simple act can build their self-esteem and reinforce positive self-talk. Another exercise is to reflect on a recent experience and how it made them feel. This helps them process their emotions and understand their reactions. Setting a personal goal for the day and repeating it while looking in the mirror can also be powerful. It gives them a clear focus and a sense of purpose. Additionally, using the mirror to practice deep breathing and calming techniques can help them manage stress and anxiety. These exercises not only promote emotional regulation but also create a moment of calm in their busy day.

As a parent, your support and encouragement are vital in making the self-reflection mirror a valuable tool for your child. Model self-reflection by sharing your own experiences and how they help you grow. For instance, you might share how you reflect on your day and the lessons you've learned. This not only sets a positive example but also shows them that self-reflection is a lifelong practice. Encourage regular use of the mirror and provide positive feedback when they share their reflections. Praise their efforts and the insights they gain, reinforcing the importance of this practice. Discussing their reflections and offering guidance when needed can also help them navigate their emotions and experiences more effectively.

INTERACTIVE ELEMENT: SELF-REFLECTION MIRROR AFFIRMATION CARDS

To enhance the self-reflection experience, you can create a set of affirmation cards to use with the mirror. These cards can include phrases like:

- "I am brave."
- "I am a good friend."
- "I can solve problems."
- "I am loved."

Encourage your child to pick a card each day, read it aloud while looking in the mirror, and reflect on what it means to them. This daily ritual can reinforce positive self-perception and provide a moment of encouragement and motivation. By integrating these affirmation cards into their routine, you can make the practice of self-reflection more engaging and impactful. It helps children internalize positive messages and build a stronger, more confident sense of self.

11.3 THOUGHT-TRACKING CHARTS

A few weeks ago, you noticed that your nine-year-old son, David, seemed more anxious than usual. He often expressed worries about school and friendships, and you could see that these negative thoughts were affecting his mood and behavior. To help David become more aware of his thought patterns and encourage positive thinking, you decided to introduce him to thought-tracking charts. Thought-tracking is a powerful tool for self-reflection, allowing children to visualize their thoughts and understand how they influence their emotions and actions. It helps them become aware of recurring negative thoughts and supports emotional regulation and problem-solving.

Creating effective thought-tracking charts is straightforward. Start with a simple template that includes columns for different types of thoughts, such as positive, negative, and neutral. Each column should have space for writing down specific thoughts and the related emotions. This visual layout makes it easier for children to categorize and analyze their thoughts. Providing examples can help your child understand how to use the chart. For instance, if

David writes, "I'm worried I won't do well on my math test," in the negative thoughts column, he can also note how this thought makes him feel anxious. On the other hand, a positive thought like, "I did well on my last test," can be linked to feelings of confidence and pride.

Using thought-tracking charts can involve several specific activities. One effective exercise is the daily thought log. Encourage your child to write down three thoughts they had during the day and how each thought made them feel. This practice not only helps them become more mindful of their thought patterns but also promotes self-awareness. Another useful activity is to challenge negative thoughts. When David writes down a negative thought, guide him to reframe it in a positive way. For example, if he writes, "I'm not good at sports," help him see a different perspective by adding, "I'm improving with practice, and I enjoy playing with my friends."

Identifying thought patterns is another valuable exercise. By tracking recurring thoughts over a week, you and your child can discuss any patterns that emerge. Maybe David frequently worries about schoolwork on Sundays, which could be linked to the upcoming week. Recognizing these patterns allows you to address specific concerns and develop strategies to cope with them. Regular review of the thought-tracking chart helps in this process. Set aside time to go through the chart together, discussing any trends or changes. Ask David how his thoughts impact his behavior and emotions. This discussion can lead to setting goals for positive thinking and self-improvement. For instance, if he notices that positive thoughts about his abilities lead to better performance, he can focus on nurturing those thoughts.

INTERACTIVE ELEMENT: WEEKLY THOUGHT-TRACKING CHART TEMPLATE

To make thought-tracking engaging, create a weekly chart template with columns for positive, negative, and neutral thoughts. Include spaces for specific thoughts and related emotions. Encourage your child to use different colors for each type of thought, making the chart visually appealing. This template can be a valuable tool for helping children like David become more aware of their thought patterns and develop healthier thinking habits. Regular use of thought-tracking charts can significantly enhance your child's ability to reflect on their thoughts, understand their emotions, and make positive changes. By integrating this practice into their routine, you support their emotional growth and resilience, helping them navigate life's challenges with greater confidence.

11.4 REFLECTION THROUGH DRAWING

Drawing can be a powerful tool for self-reflection, especially for children who may find it easier to express their thoughts and emotions visually rather than verbally. When children draw, they engage in a creative and non-verbal form of self-expression that allows them to explore their inner world in a unique way. This process encourages introspection, helping them to visualize their feelings and experiences. It can be particularly calming and therapeutic, providing a soothing outlet for emotions that might otherwise be difficult to articulate.

To create effective reflection drawing activities, start by using prompts that encourage children to draw their feelings or experiences. These prompts should be open-ended to allow for a wide range of interpretations and creativity. Providing a variety of drawing materials, such as crayons, markers, and colored pencils, can make the activity more engaging and enjoyable. It's also important to create a supportive and non-judgmental environment where children feel free to express themselves without fear of criticism. This safe space encourages them to be honest and open in their drawings.

Specific prompts can guide children in their reflection drawings. For example, asking them to "Draw a picture of your favorite memory from today" helps them focus on positive experiences and recall details that made the day special. Another prompt, like "Create a drawing that represents how you feel right now," allows them to explore their current emotional state visually. This can be particularly helpful for children who struggle to put their feelings into words. Encouraging them to "Illustrate a time when you felt proud of yourself" helps them recognize and celebrate their achievements, boosting their self-esteem. Lastly, "Draw a picture of your goals and dreams for the future" inspires them to think about their aspirations and motivates them to work towards their goals.

Discussing and sharing these drawings can deepen the reflective process. Ask open-ended questions about the drawings and their meanings, such as "What made you choose those colors?" or "What does this part of the drawing represent?" These questions encourage children to think more deeply about their artwork and the feelings behind it. Encourage them to share their drawings with a trusted adult or peer, fostering a sense of connection and understanding. Using the drawings as a starting point for deeper discussions about thoughts and feelings can provide valuable insights and strengthen the parent-child bond.

Incorporating reflection through drawing into your child's routine can be a rewarding and insightful practice. By providing the right prompts, materials, and environment, you can help your child explore their emotions and experiences in a fun, creative, and meaningful way. This practice not only enhances their self-awareness but also provides a therapeutic outlet for their feelings, contributing to their overall emotional well-being.

In the next chapter, we will discuss the crucial role of parental involvement and support in helping children develop these essential executive functioning skills.

Activity Worksheet

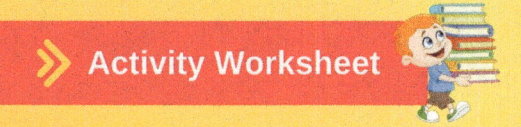

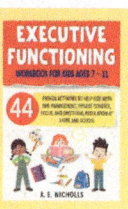

Chapter 11 — Self-Reflection

Activity: Daily Journaling Prompts

- Name : _____
- Date : _____

Daily Journal Prompts

Choose one or more of these prompts to reflect on your day. Use them to explore your thoughts and feelings!

1. **What made you smile today?**

   ----

2. **Describe a time when you felt proud of yourself.**

   ----

3. **What is something you want to improve on?**

   ----

4. **Write/tell me about a fun activity you did today.**

   ----

5. **What is something kind you did for someone else today?**

   ----

6. **What is a challenge you faced today?**

   ----

7. **What is something new you learned today?**

   ----

8. **What is one thing you are grateful for today?**

   ----

9. **What is something that made you feel calm or peaceful today?**

   ----

10. **What is one goal you have for tomorrow?**

Activity Worksheet

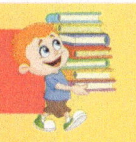

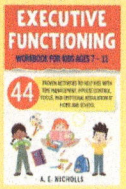

Chapter 11 — Self-Reflection

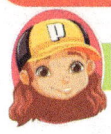

Activity: The Self-Reflection Mirror

Affirmation Cards for Mirror Time

Encourage your child to pick one affirmation card each day, read it aloud while looking in the mirror, and reflect on what it means to them. These cards help boost self-esteem, positivity, and self-confidence.

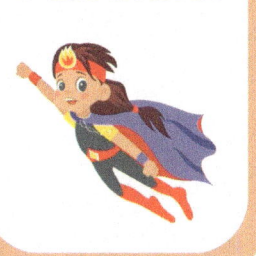

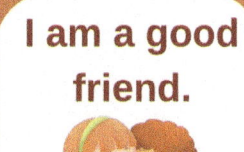

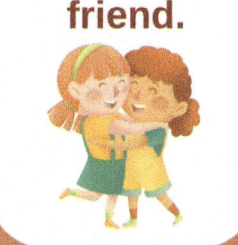

- I am brave.
- I am a good friend.
- I can solve problems.
- I am loved.
- I am strong.
- I am kind.
- I believe in myself.
- I can learn from my mistakes.
- I am creative.

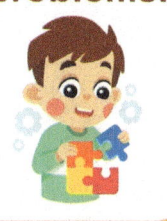

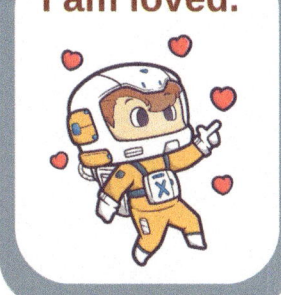

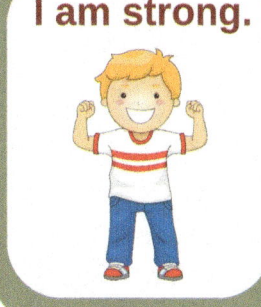

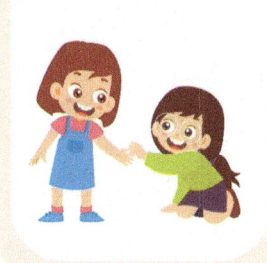

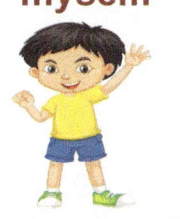

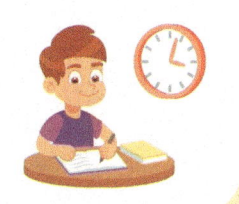

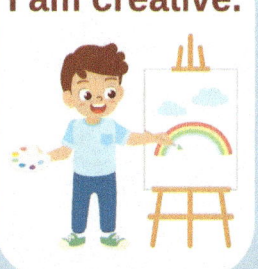

Activity Worksheet

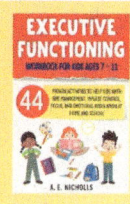

Chapter 11 — Self-Reflection

Activity: Thought-Tracking Charts

- **Name :** _____
- **Week of :** _____

Instructions:

Each day, write down your thoughts and the emotions that go with them. Use different colors to make it fun!
- **Positive thoughts:** Use a bright color (e.g., green, blue)
- **Negative thoughts:** Use a darker color (e.g., red, black)
- **Neutral thoughts:** Use a soft color (e.g., gray, yellow)

Day	Positive Thoughts (Bright colors)	Emotion	Negative Thoughts (Dark colors)	Emotion	Neutral Thoughts (Soft colors)	Emotion
Monday						
Tuesday						
Wednesday						
Thursday						
Friday						
Saturday						
Sunday						

5. Reflection Section:

1. What types of thoughts did you have the most of this week?

   ----

2. How did your positive thoughts make you feel?

   ----

3. How did you handle your negative thoughts?
   ----

4. How can you have more positive or neutral thoughts next week?

Activity Worksheet

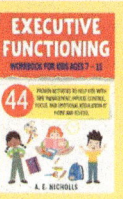

Chapter 11 — **Self-Reflection**

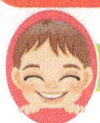

Activity: Reflection Through Drawing

- Name : _____
- Date : _____

Drawing Prompts
- Draw a picture of your favorite memory from today.
- Create a drawing that represents how you feel right now.
- Illustrate a time when you felt proud of yourself.
- Draw a picture of your goals and dreams for the future.

Reflection Section:

- What made you choose those colors?

- What does this part of the drawing represent?

- How did you feel while creating this drawing?

- What do you want to remember about this drawing?

12

PARENTAL INVOLVEMENT AND SUPPORT

"Parental involvement is the cornerstone of a child's development, fostering a nurturing environment where children can thrive emotionally, socially, and academically. Through shared activities and open communication, parents can build strong, supportive relationships that last a lifetime."

— DR. KENNETH R. GINSBURG

On a lazy Sunday afternoon, you might find eleven-year-old Sam and his dad, Michael, in the garage, engrossed in building a birdhouse. It's not just about hammering nails and fitting pieces together; it's about the stories shared, the jokes cracked, and the lessons learned along the way. This simple activity becomes a treasured memory, a bonding experience that leaves a lasting impact on both Sam and Michael. Spending quality time with your child through structured activities offers immense benefits, fostering a strong parent-child bond while providing opportunities for learning and development.

12.1 PARENT-CHILD ACTIVITY TIME

Engaging in structured activities together enhances your relationship with your child, creating a foundation of trust and open communication. These moments provide a platform for discussing thoughts, feelings, and experiences in a relaxed setting, away from the pressures of daily routines. This not only strengthens your bond but also builds a sense of security and support for your child, knowing they have a dependable and loving presence in their life. Moreover, these shared experiences encourage mutual learning and development as both you and your child explore new skills and interests together.

When selecting activities to do with your child, it's important to consider their interests and preferences. Choose activities that align with what they enjoy, whether it's cooking, crafting, or exploring nature. This ensures that they remain engaged and enthusiastic. Including both indoor and outdoor options keeps the experiences diverse and refreshing. Strive for a balance between fun and educational value, incorporating activities that promote executive functioning skills, such as planning, organizing, and problem-solving. For instance, cooking together can teach your child about following instructions, measuring ingredients, and understanding the importance of timing.

Some specific activities that you can do together include cooking or baking a new recipe. This not only teaches practical life skills but also provides a platform for discussing nutrition, measurements, and even cultural traditions. Building a DIY project or craft can be incredibly rewarding, as it involves planning, creativity, and patience. Whether it's assembling a model, creating a scrapbook, or constructing a birdhouse like Sam and Michael, these projects offer a sense of accomplishment and pride. Playing board games that require strategy and teamwork fosters critical thinking, cooperation, and healthy competition. Games like chess, checkers, or cooperative board games can be both fun and educational. Exploring nature through hiking or gardening allows you to connect with the environment, learn about plants and wildlife, and enjoy physical activity together.

To maximize the benefits of parent-child activity time, set aside regular, uninterrupted periods dedicated to these activities. Consistency is key, as it reinforces the importance of these moments and helps establish a routine. Encourage active participation and collaboration, allowing your child to take the lead or make decisions whenever possible. This fosters independence and confidence. Use this time to discuss thoughts, feelings, and experiences, creating an open dialogue that strengthens your bond. Celebrate successes, no matter how small, and enjoy the process together. The journey is often more significant than the outcome, and the memories created during these activities will be cherished for years to come.

REFLECTION SECTION: ACTIVITY JOURNAL

Maintaining an activity journal can enhance the experience. After each activity, encourage your child to jot down their thoughts, what they enjoyed, and what they learned. This not only reinforces the learning experience but also provides a keepsake of shared memories. Include prompts like "What was your favorite part of today's activity?" or "What new skill did you learn?" Reviewing this journal together can be a delightful way to reflect on your time spent together and plan future activities based on your child's interests and reflections.

12.2 CO-PLANNING WEEKLY SCHEDULES

Imagine the start of a busy week. Your child, Umber, is juggling school assignments, soccer practice, and piano lessons. Instead of feeling overwhelmed, she feels in control because she co-planned her weekly schedule with you. Co-planning schedules not only teaches time management but also fosters a sense of responsibility and independence. When children take part in organizing their time, they learn to prioritize tasks and allocate their energy effectively. This collaboration enhances communication and strengthens the bond between you and your child, making them feel valued and heard.

To get started, sit down together at the beginning of the week. This can become a regular Sunday evening ritual where you both discuss the upcoming tasks, events, and activities. Lay everything out on the table—school assignments, extracurricular activities, family events, and any other commitments. By discussing these together, you help your child understand the importance of planning and the need to balance various responsibilities. Prioritize the tasks and allocate time for each one, ensuring that the most important activities are given the attention they need. This process not only teaches your child how to manage their time but also instills a sense of control and ownership over their schedule.

Once you have discussed and prioritized the tasks, create a visual schedule that is easy to follow. This could be a planner, a calendar, or even a large chart on the wall. Use different colors for different types of activities—school tasks in blue, chores in green, and leisure activities in red. For younger children, visual aids like stickers or drawings can make the schedule more engaging and easier to understand. This visual representation helps your child see their week at a glance, making it easier to stay organized and on track.

There are several tools and resources that can aid in co-planning weekly schedules. Planners and calendars are traditional yet effective tools for organizing tasks. Scheduling apps can also be useful, especially those that allow for color coding and reminders. These digital tools can be accessed from anywhere, making it easy to update and review the schedule on the go. For younger children, consider using visual aids like stickers, drawings, or even magnetic boards where they can move task pieces around. Physically touching the schedule can make the planning process more engaging and enjoyable.

Regularly reviewing and adjusting the schedule is key to its success. Schedule a mid-week check-in to assess how things are going. Are there tasks that took longer than expected? Are there new commitments that need to be added? Be flexible and open to changes as needed.

This adaptability teaches your child that while planning is important, it's also essential to be able to adjust when things don't go as planned. Reflect on what worked well and what could be improved. Encourage your child to take an active role in updating the schedule, fostering a sense of responsibility and independence.

By involving your child in the co-planning of their weekly schedule, you are not only teaching them valuable life skills but also creating a collaborative environment where they feel empowered. The skills they learn through this process—time management, prioritization, and flexibility—will serve them well throughout their lives.

12.3 FAMILY GOAL SETTING

Setting family goals can be a transformative practice, bringing everyone closer together. Imagine your family sitting around the dining table, each person sharing their dreams and aspirations. This moment of unity and teamwork fosters a sense of collective purpose. When you set goals as a family, you create an environment of mutual support and accountability. Each member feels connected to a shared objective, whether it's planning a vacation, starting a new hobby, or undertaking a home improvement project. This collective effort not only strengthens family bonds but also teaches your children the value of goal-setting and achievement. They learn that working together, supporting each other, and celebrating successes are essential elements of personal and communal growth.

To set family goals effectively, begin by gathering everyone for a goal-setting session. This can be a special family meeting where each person gets a chance to voice their ideas and aspirations. Encourage a brainstorming session where all potential goals are discussed openly. Ensure that everyone feels heard and valued in this process. After brainstorming, choose goals that are meaningful and achievable for everyone. It's important to select objectives that resonate with the whole family, ensuring that each member is invested in the outcome. Once you have chosen your goals, break them down into actionable steps and assign responsibilities. This division of tasks promotes a sense of ownership and accountability, making each person feel like part of the journey.

For example, planning a family vacation can be a delightful goal. Discuss potential destinations, research activities, and allocate tasks such as booking accommodations, planning the itinerary, and budgeting for the trip. Another goal might be completing a home improvement project together, like creating a garden or redecorating a room. This not only beautifies your living space but also provides opportunities for teamwork and creativity. Starting a new family tradition or hobby, such as a weekly game night or a monthly cooking challenge, can bring joy and consistency to your family life. Volunteering or participating in community service as a family is another excellent goal. It instills values of empathy and social responsibility, teaching your children the importance of giving back to the community.

Tracking progress and celebrating achievements are important parts of the goal-setting process. Use a goal chart or journal to record your progress. This visual representation helps everyone stay focused and motivated. Schedule regular check-ins to discuss how the goals are going. These sessions provide opportunities to reflect on what's working well and what might need adjustment. Celebrate milestones and successes with a family reward or activity. Whether it's a special dinner, a movie night, or a day out, these celebrations reinforce the positive outcomes of working together. Reflecting on the journey and what was learned along the way is equally important. Discuss the challenges faced, the solutions found, and the personal growth experienced by each family member. This reflection not only acknowledges the hard work and dedication but also sets the stage for future goal-setting.

12.4 JOINT REFLECTION SESSIONS

Joint reflection sessions offer a unique opportunity for families to come together and share their experiences, thoughts, and feelings. Imagine sitting in the living room, everyone gathered comfortably, sharing stories about the week's highs and lows. This practice encourages open communication and emotional sharing, creating a safe space where everyone feels heard and valued. It provides opportunities for mutual support and understanding, helping family members connect on a deeper level. Reflecting together helps identify areas for improvement and growth, reinforcing positive behaviors and achievements. It teaches children that self-reflection is a valuable tool for personal development and fosters a culture of continuous improvement within the family.

To conduct effective reflection sessions, schedule regular, dedicated time for this activity. Weekly family meetings are ideal, as they provide a consistent opportunity for everyone to come together and reflect. Create a safe and supportive environment for sharing, where each person feels comfortable expressing their thoughts and feelings without fear of judgment. Use structured prompts or questions to guide the discussion, ensuring that the conversation remains focused and meaningful. Encourage active listening and respectful communication, teaching your children the importance of empathy and understanding.

Prompts can help facilitate these discussions. Ask questions like, "What was the highlight of your week and why?" to encourage sharing of positive experiences. "What challenges did you face, and how did you overcome them?" helps identify areas for growth and resilience. "What are you grateful for this week?" fosters a sense of gratitude and positivity. "What goals do you have for the coming week?" encourages forward-thinking and planning.

Using reflection sessions for continuous improvement involves discussing areas for growth and setting new goals or adjustments. Celebrate successes and recognize efforts, reinforcing the importance of acknowledging achievements. Ensure that everyone feels heard and valued during the sessions, creating an inclusive environment where each person's contributions are appreciated. This practice not only strengthens family bonds but also teaches children the importance of reflection and continuous improvement.

As you engage in these joint reflection sessions, you'll find that they become a cherished family tradition, a time to connect, support, and grow together. This practice helps build a strong foundation of communication and understanding, equipping your

Activity Worksheet

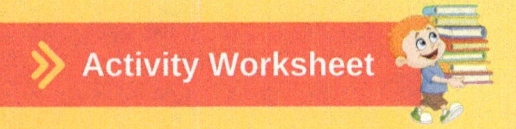

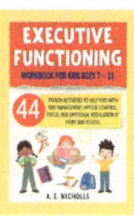

Chapter 12 — Parental Involvement & Support

Activity: Parent-Child Activity Time

- Name : _____
- Date : _____

Today's Activity

- **What did you do today?**

(Cooking, crafting, exploring nature, etc.)

Examples of Activities

Cooking: Bake cookies, make a pizza, or create a fruit salad.
Crafting: Paint, build with clay, or make a scrapbook.
Exploring Nature: Go on a nature walk, collect leaves, or plant seeds.

Journal Prompts

1. What was your favorite part of today's activity?
----

2. What new skill did you learn?
----

3. What did you enjoy the most about this activity?
----

4. Was there something that was challenging? How did you overcome it?
----

5. What do you want to do differently next time?

Reflection Section:

- What did you learn from today's activity?

- How did this activity make you feel?

- Would you like to do this activity again? Why or why not?

Activity Worksheet

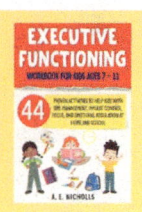

Chapter 12 — Parental Involvement & Support

Activity: Co-Planning Weekly Schedules

- **Name :** _____
- **Week of :** _____

Scheduled Activities for the Week

Day	Activity	Time	Supplies Needed
Monday			
Tuesday			
Wednesday			
Thursday			
Friday			
Saturday			
Sunday			

Examples of Activities

Monday: Bake cookies together
Tuesday: Crafting time (make a paper collage)
Wednesday: Nature walk and collect leaves
Thursday: Build a puzzle or play a board game
Friday: Movie night or reading together
Saturday: Visit the park or go for a bike ride
Sunday: Make a scrapbook of the week's activities

Joint Reflection Area

- What did we enjoy most about our time together?

- What was our favorite activity and why?

- What did we learn from our activities this week?

- What do we want to plan for next week?

Activity Worksheet

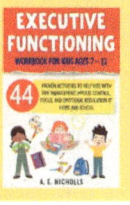

Chapter 12 — Parental Involvement & Support

Activity: Family Goal Setting

Family Goal

(Write down the goal your family wants to achieve. It can be big or small!)

Goal : _____

Progress Tracker

- (Mark your progress toward the goal each week!)

Week	Tasks Completed	How Did We Work Together?
Week 1		
Week 2		
Week 3		
Week 4		

Reflection & Celebration

- **What decision did you make today? What did we enjoy the most while working on our goal?**
  _____
  _____

- **What challenges did we face, and how did we overcome them?**
  _____
  _____

- **How did we work as a team?**
  _____
  _____

- **How will we celebrate our achievement?**
  _____
  _____

Activity Worksheet

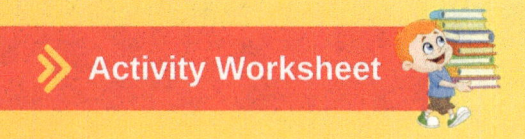

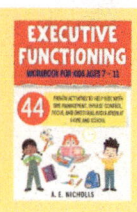

Chapter 12 — Parental Involvement & Support

Activity: Joint Reflection Sessions

- **Name :** _____
- **Week of :** _____

Weekly Highlights & Challenges

- (Each family member shares their favorite moment of the week and a challenge they faced.)

Family Member	Highlight of the Week	Challenge	How I Handled It

Family Support

- (How did we support each other this week?)

What Did We Learn About Each Other?

- (Share something new we discovered about each other during this reflection time.)

Goals for Next Week

- (Discuss something the family can work on together or individually for the upcoming week.)

AFTERWORD

"Every step you take in supporting your child's development, no matter how small, is a step toward unlocking their fullest potential. Your dedication and love are the greatest gifts you can offer them."

— DR. JANE NELSEN

As we reach the end of this book, let's take a moment to reflect on the journey we've shared. From understanding executive functioning to implementing practical strategies and working on activities, we've explored numerous ways to support your child's development. Each chapter was aimed to equip you with tools and activities that are designed to make everyday challenges more manageable and to facilitate growth in key areas.

We've discussed the importance of executive functioning skills, such as time management, impulse control, focus, and emotional regulation. Through engaging activities like the Hidden Object Concentration Game and the Freeze Game, we've seen how these skills can be built in fun and interactive ways. We've also delved into creating daily routines, setting goals, and using visual aids, all aimed at helping your child thrive both at home and school.

One of the key takeaways from this book is the power of practical, hands-on activities. These activities make learning fun and effective. Whether it's through focused breathing exercises to enhance concentration or memory-matching games to boost recall, each activity serves a purpose. They aren't just tasks to complete but opportunities for your child to develop essential life skills.

Another important point is the role of parents. Your engagement and support are crucial. By co-planning schedules, setting family goals, and spending quality time together, you create a nurturing environment. This environment encourages your child to practice and apply the skills they are learning. Your presence and participation make a significant difference in your child's growth and confidence.

Now, let's think about the call to action. I encourage you to take the strategies and activities discussed and integrate them into your daily routines. Start small, choose a few activities that resonate most with your child's needs, and build from there. Consistency is key. Regular practice will reinforce these skills and make them a natural part of your child's behavior.

Remember, progress might be gradual, and that's okay. Celebrate small victories and acknowledge the effort your child puts into each task. Be patient and persistent, and provide positive reinforcement. Your support and encouragement are the foundation of their success.

As a pediatric occupational therapist, I've seen firsthand the incredible impact that dedication and targeted activities can have on a child's development. I've witnessed children transform their struggles into strengths, and I've seen families grow closer through shared efforts and achievements. You have the power to make a lasting difference in your child's life.

In closing, I want to leave you with an inspirational message. Every child has the potential to overcome challenges and achieve their fullest potential. Believe in your child's abilities and trust in the process. Your unwavering support and the strategies we've discussed will pave the way for their success.

Thank you for allowing me to be a part of your journey. Remember, every step you take, no matter how small, is a step toward a brighter future for your child. Keep striving, keep believing, and together, let's help your child shine.

A FINAL NOTE OF GRATITUDE

"It is easier to build strong children than to repair broken men."

— FREDERICK DOUGLASS

We've reached the end of our exploration into enhancing executive functioning skills, but in many ways, this is just the beginning of your journey with your child. The activities, strategies, and insights shared in this book are tools that will continue to serve you and your child for years to come.

If you've found value in this book, I would be deeply appreciative if you could take a few minutes to leave a review. Your words have the power to guide other parents who are seeking ways to support their children's executive functioning skills.

Thank you for allowing me to be a part of your family's journey. Your dedication to your child's growth is making a real difference, and I'm honored to have played a small role in that process.

Remember, every step forward, no matter how small, is a victory. Keep believing in your child and in yourself. Together, we're nurturing the next generation of capable, confident individuals.

With heartfelt gratitude,

A. E. Nicholls

BIBLIOGRAPHY

American Academy of Pediatrics. (n.d.). Breathing exercises for kids. Children's Health. https://www.childrens.com/health-wellness/breathing-exercises-for-kids

Babbitt, F. C. (Trans.). (1927). Moralia. Harvard University Press. (Original work published c. 100 AD)

Covey, S. R. (1989). The 7 habits of highly effective people: Powerful lessons in personal change. Free Press.

Dawson, P. (2012). Smart but scattered: The revolutionary "executive skills" approach to helping kids reach their potential. The Guilford Press.

Day, D. (2012). Be happy now! Become the active director of your life. CreateSpace Independent Publishing Platform.

Duckworth, A. L., Gendler, T. S., & Gross, J. J. (2014). Self-control in school-age children. Educational Psychologist, 49(3), 199-217. https://doi.org/10.1080/00461520.2014.926225

Ginsburg, K. R. (2007). Building resilience in children and teens: Giving kids roots and wings. American Academy of Pediatrics.

Glen, S. (2019). Teaching children problem-solving skills. Journal of Educational Psychology, 111(2), 201-213. https://doi.org/10.1037/edu0000322

Goleman, D. (2013). Focus: The hidden driver of excellence. Harper.

Huebner, E. S. (2001). Manual for the multidimensional students' life satisfaction scale. University of South Carolina.

Joubert, J. (1842). Pensees. P. Jannet.

Keeshan, B. (2004). Good morning, captain: 50 wonderful years with Bob Keeshan, TV's Captain Kangaroo. Fairview Press.

Nelsen, J. (2006). Positive discipline. Ballantine Books.

Siegel, D. J., & Bryson, T. P. (2011). The whole-brain child: 12 revolutionary strategies to nurture your child's developing mind. Delacorte Press.

Websites and Online Resources:

ADDitude. (n.d.). Executive function disorder in children. https://www.additudemag.com/executive-function-disorder-in-children-symptoms/

All Round Club. (n.d.). The importance of teamwork for children: A guide to building collaborative skills. https://allroundclub.com/blog/the-importance-of-teamwork-for-children-a-guide-to-building-collaborative-skills/

A Touch of Class Teaching. (n.d.). 20 examples of SMART goals for students and fun growth mindset posters. https://www.atouchofclassteaching.com/20-examples-of-smart-goals-for-students-and-fun-growth-mindset-posters/

Child Mind Institute. (n.d.). Helping kids who struggle with executive functions. https://childmind.org/article/helping-kids-who-struggle-with-executive-functions/

Child Mind Institute. (n.d.). Helping kids with flexible thinking. https://childmind.org/article/helping-kids-with-flexible-thinking/

Childhood101. (n.d.). 10 kids memory games to help improve short-term memory. https://childhood101.com/short-term-memory-games/

Empowered Parents. (n.d.). 12 visual memory games and activities for kids. https://empoweredparents.co/visual-memory-games/

Empowered Parents. (n.d.). 13 benefits of puzzles for child development. https://empoweredparents.co/benefits-of-puzzles/

Everyday Speech. (n.d.). Understanding the importance of teaching creative problem solving in elementary schools. https://everydayspeech.com/blog-posts/general/understanding-the-importance-of-teaching-creative-problem-solving-in-elementary-schools/

Fun and Function. (n.d.). Simon Says: Use coordination to focus & attend. https://funandfunction.com/blog/simon-says-use-coordination-to-focus-attend

GetGoally. (n.d.). Kid-friendly time management tools for neurodiverse learners. https://getgoally.com/blog/time-management-tools/

Harvard Health Publishing. (2020, December 16). Executive function in children: Why it matters and how to help. https://www.health.harvard.edu/blog/executive-function-in-children-why-it-matters-and-how-to-help-2020121621583

Instructables. (n.d.). Calm bottle (aka glitter jar): 3 steps. https://www.instructables.com/Calm-Bottle-aka-Glitter-Jar/

Johnson, L. B. (n.d.). *Lady Bird Johnson quotes.* BrainyQuote. Retrieved from https://www.brainyquote.com/quotes/lady_bird_johnson_150168

Learnfully. (n.d.). Supporting K-12 learners: The importance of executive functioning skills. https://learnfully.com/state-of-neurodiversity-2023-report/

Mental Health Center Kids. (n.d.). 10 teaching patience activities for kids. https://mentalhealthcenterkids.com/blogs/articles/teaching-patience-activities

Mindful Mazing. (n.d.). 44 powerful problem solving activities for kids. https://www.mindfulmazing.com/problem-solving-activities-for-kids/

My Good Brain. (n.d.). Why is self-reflection important in children? https://www.mygoodbrain.org/blog/why-is-self-reflection-important-in-children

National Center for Biotechnology Information. (n.d.). Executive functioning heterogeneity in pediatric ADHD. https://www.ncbi.nlm.nih.gov/pmc/articles/PMC6204311/

National Center for Biotechnology Information. (n.d.). Executive functioning and neurodevelopmental disorders in early childhood: A prospective study. https://www.ncbi.nlm.nih.gov/pmc/articles/PMC6805591/

Parents. (n.d.). The right way to set up a reward system for kids. https://www.parents.com/toddlers-preschoolers/discipline/the-right-way-to-set-up-a-reward-system-for-kids/

Parent.com. (2017). The importance of setting family goals – and how to do it. https://www.parent.com/blogs/conversations/2017-the-importance-of-setting-family-goals-and-how-to-do-it

PBS. (n.d.). 7 activities that help kids communicate with others. https://www.pbs.org/parents/thrive/7-activities-that-help-kids-communicate-with-others

Scholastic. (n.d.). The age-by-age guide to teaching kids time management. https://www.scholastic.com/parents/family-life/parent-child/teach-kids-to-manage-time.html

ScienceDirect. (n.d.). Executive functioning in children with ASD + ADHD and ASD + ADHD symptoms. https://www.sciencedirect.com/science/article/abs/pii/S1750946721000829

SplashLearn. (n.d.). 15 best concentration games for kids to improve their focus. https://www.splashlearn.com/blog/concentration-games-for-kids/

Study.com. (n.d.). Behavior chart for kids | Overview, benefits & examples. https://study.com/academy/lesson/how-to-use-a-behavior-chart-effectively.html

Study.com. (n.d.). Brainstorming techniques lesson for kids. https://study.com/academy/lesson/brainstorming-techniques-lesson-for-kids.html

Taste of Home. (n.d.). 55 recipes to teach your kids right now. https://www.tasteofhome.com/collection/recipes-to-teach-your-kids-right-now/

The Many Little Joys. (n.d.). A simple chore system for kids that really works! {+ free printable chore chart}. https://themanylittlejoys.com/a-simple-chore-system-for-kids-that-really-works-free-printable-chore-chart/

The OT Toolbox. (n.d.). Self-reflection activities. https://www.theottoolbox.com/self-reflection-activities-for-kids/

The Pathway 2 Success. (n.d.). 25 self-control activities for children. https://www.thepathway2success.com/25-self-control-activities-for-children/

Understood. (n.d.). A day in the life of a child with executive function challenges. https://www.understood.org/en/articles/a-day-in-the-life-of-a-child-with-executive-functioning-issues

Understood. (n.d.). Social situations to role-play with your child in different grades. https://www.understood.org/en/articles/social-situations-to-role-play-with-your-child-in-different-grades

Understood. (n.d.). What is executive function? https://www.understood.org/en/articles/what-is-executive-function

Waterford.org. (n.d.). 51 mindfulness exercises for kids in the classroom. https://www.waterford.org/resources/mindfulnes-activities-for-kids/

We Are Teachers. (n.d.). 80+ journal prompts for kids for creativity & self-discovery. https://blog.gratefulness.me/journal-prompts-for-kids/

California State University, Northridge. (n.d.). 10 tips for using co-planning time more efficiently. https://www.csun.edu/sites/default/files/10-Tips-for-Using-Co-Planning-Time-More-Efficiently.pdf

ALSO BY A. E. NICHOLLS

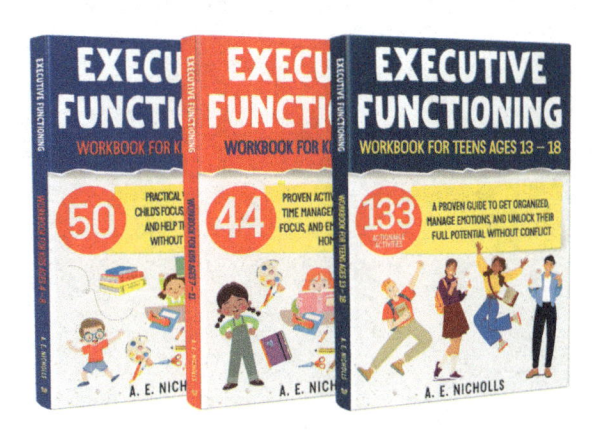

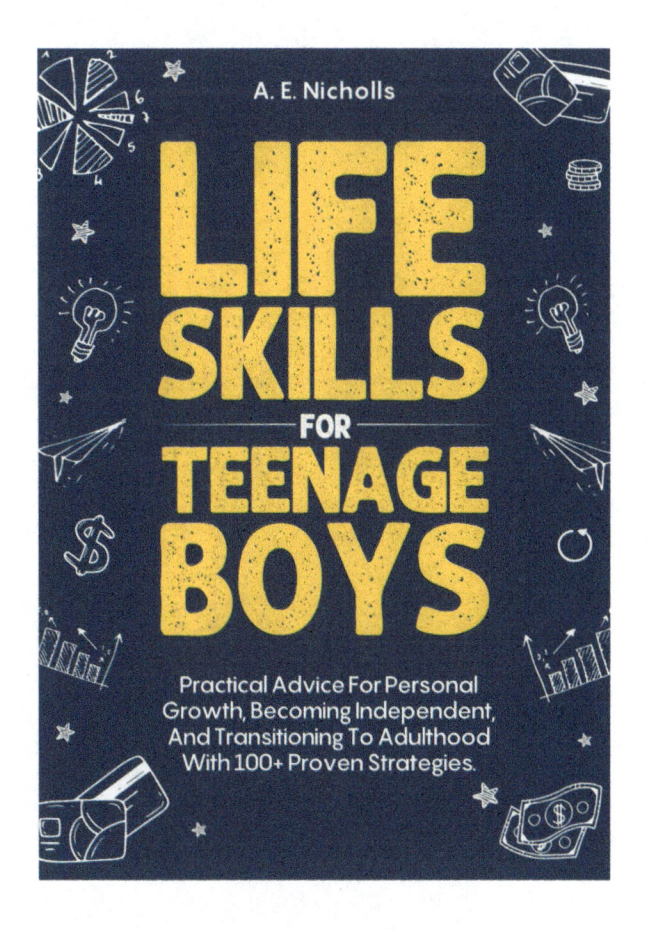

EXECUTIVE FUNCTIONING WORKBOOK FOR KIDS AGES 4 – 8
EXECUTIVE FUNCTIONING WORKBOOK FOR KIDS AGES 7 – 11
EXECUTIVE FUNCTIONING WORKBOOK FOR TEENS, AGES 13 - 18
LIFE SKILLS FOR TEENAGE BOOKS

Made in the USA
Monee, IL
25 January 2025